YOUR
HEALTHY
CHILD

ALICE LIKOWSKI DUNCAN, D.C.

YOUR HEALTHY CHILD

A GUIDE TO NATURAL HEALTH CARE FOR CHILDREN

JEREMY P. TARCHER, INC.
Los Angeles

For T.F., with Love

Although the natural medicines offered in this book are generally safe, it is impossible to predict an individual's reaction to a particular treatment. If in doubt about a remedy or a child's reaction, we encourage you to consult a qualified physician or practitioner of natural medicine. Neither the author nor the publisher accept responsibility for any effects that may occur from any treatment included in this book.

Library of Congress Cataloging-in-Publication Data

Likowski Duncan, Alice.
    Your healthy child : a guide to natural health for children / Alice Likowski Duncan ; foreword by Lendon Smith.
        p.   cm.
    ISBN 0-87477-619-8 (cl.)
    ISBN 0-87477-620-1 (pbk.)
    1. Pediatrics—Popular works. 2. Naturopathy. 3. Children—diseases—Alternative treatment.   I. Title
    RJ47.L65   1990   90-19848
    625.5 ' 42—dc20   CIP

Jeremy P. Tarcher, Inc.
5858 Wilshire Blvd., Suite 200
Los Angeles, CA 90036

Distributed by St. Martin's Press, New York

Design by Susan Shankin

Manufactured in the United States of America
10 9 8 7 6 5 4 3 2 1

First Edition

CONTENTS

ACKNOWLEDGMENTS

I would like to thank the late Faredoon Driver, who introduced me to homeopathic medicine, and also Dr. Ghani—whom I never met, but whose life and antics have cheered me in taxing and unpredictable times. Their tenacity, strength, flexibility, honesty and astonishing adherence to their own personalities have been an inspiration. I also thank their boss and childhood friend, whoever he is.

Special appreciation and love go to my son, Doonie, who is sweet and imaginative and a great pal. Thanks to H.C. de R. for making apple pies, taking my soliloquies seriously, and trying to fix the rollercoaster. Thanks to the IFH gang, and all physicians and practitioners who try to do no harm. Thanks to Lois for wanting this book and suggesting that I write it. Thanks to my parents, my good friends Harry, Eruch, Elizabeth, Renee, John, Evan, Laura, Doug, Marnie, Paul, Judy, Carl, Sophie, and Tess, the families who have tested (and been tested by?) this book, and to my patients— who cheerfully adapt to my weird writing schedule.

Tremendous gratitude to Donna Zerner, my editor, whose lucid mind and talent for organization have enriched the matter of this book and combed out many snarls. Her help in completing the final manuscript has been a great relief, and admirable.

FOREWORD

Books on child care, especially child *health* care, are difficult to write. One needs to be as inclusive as possible, without being overwhelming. A pneumonia can appear no more serious than the flu that is going around. At what point does a parent stop and say, "Help, I'm over my head"?

A book on home care must be comforting and helpful; the information has to be clear and useful, simple and direct. The author must assume the role of the scientific grandmother, giving the parents safe and helpful things to do while they wait for the child's natural defense mechanisms to get the child well.

Alice Duncan has avoided the pitfalls of medical how-to writing, and I applaud her. She has successfully included—in a reasonable, understandable form—just about everything modern parents need to know about the diagnosis and natural treatment of childhood illnesses. The descriptions of the illnesses and their treatment are short, accurate, and exude confidence. One has the feeling that if Dr. Duncan says something will work, it will. And, also important, she allows that medical or allopathic doctors have their place in the care of the sick.

Alice Duncan is raising her voice for conservatism in the treatment of children because she has seen the problems that can arise when sick children are overtreated with "standard" medicines instead of being helped by an inexpensive, safe, natural remedy. She is trying to help modern parents experience the joy of caring more completely for their children. Love is not enough. Parents want to know—and *need* to know—how to practice safe treatment, and how to use preventive methods so their child will not get sick again.

This book is practical and the methods are safe. Parents should have it and its remedies by their bedside.

—LENDON SMITH, M.D.

PART 1
INFORMATION

Introduction

For the past twenty years, I have used natural remedies on myself, friends, patients and children, with gratifying results. Natural healing techniques are often labeled "alternative" medicine, but I prefer to regard them as "traditional," since—for most of human history—people have turned to natural remedies to treat disease and injury.

During the last century, interventionist and often toxic medical methods such as the use of chemical drugs and high-tech procedures became the dominant mode of practice. As the scientific approach to health care grew more abstruse and complex, people became dependent on doctors, thinking themselves unable to understand and promote their own health. In the last few decades, however, the unhealthy, often dangerous, consequences of such an attitude have become more apparent, and some of us have taken health care back into our own hands. Many people are now aware of the benefits of simple preventive techniques to encourage health, and are choosing safe and effective natural remedies for the treatment of disease.

As a chiropractic physician and natural health practitioner, I have always encouraged the use of noninvasive natural remedies and procedures that bolster the body's resources and help to prevent or overcome illness. Yet, ten years ago, when my son was born and had his first illness, like any new parent I underwent a lot of distress and uncertainty. One midnight, at the age of seven weeks, he woke up crying, with a very high fever. I was worried. I knew that fever is the body's efficient method of fighting infection, but I also knew that fever in a tiny baby can be a sign of something very serious, in which case seeing a medical doctor might be important. I *also* knew that an M.D.'s thorough attempt at diagnosis might lead to blood tests, lumbar punctures, biopsies, antibiotics "to cover the bases"—procedures I did not want my baby subjected to.

What could I do? My mind raced with doubts and fears: If my son had a viral flu that only rest would cure, how could the strain and exhaustion of all these procedures help him get well? If they gave him medication, what if he had a reaction? What if the spinal tap had complications? What if he caught meningitis from someone in the waiting room?

As a mother (and rational person), I had an aversion to dragging a feverish infant out in the night to be handled by strangers, poked with needles, and given drugs. And yet I was caught in the parent's dilemma: I wanted to do what was best for my child, but also knew if we didn't consult an M.D., I'd be blamed by the world (and myself) if something went wrong. I tried to think through the problem clearly. What did we need here? Something to help the baby overcome his illness; something the doctors didn't offer, something natural and something safe that really *worked*.

Since my teens, I had studied wild plants and herbal medicine. At twenty, my college writing studies took me to India, where I met a towering, growly, white-haired homeopath. I was intrigued by the way he chose his remedies: based on observation of his patients' specific symptoms, he cured them of roaring fevers, crippling pains, and ghastly diarrheas. Years later, I enrolled in a chiropractic school. In the bookstore there, I found and bought a book on homeopathy. In whatever shreds of spare time I had between anatomy labs, pathology tests, X ray readings, and clinic patients, I poked about in this book and advised myself to study it. I ordered some remedies through the mail, and used them on myself, my husband, my friends. But once I'd started practice (*and* had a baby!) free time became an utter luxury and I didn't return to the book. That midnight, holding my screaming infant, I knew that the time had come to pick it up again.

I observed my son. He was wailing, mouth wide open. I could see that his throat wasn't red. I gently massaged and moved his ears; he continued to cry but no specific pain was apparent. His cheeks were flushed, especially the right; he was shrieking as if outraged and angry; his fever was high, his skin was hot; he would avidly nurse for a moment, then pull away. He was only calm when I carried him briskly from room to room.

I paced around the house, then bounced him on my shoulder while I madly paged through the homeopathy book. I found a description of his symptoms under the remedy *Chamomilla*. I tapped out several pellets, dissolved them in water, and gave him a dose from a dropper. He tasted the drops and stopped screaming. He started nursing. His fever went up a bit and lasted half the night—but his sleep was restful; he didn't cry. He was happy and well in the morning. And so was I.

I had dealt in a positive way with my child's illness, and hadn't been pushed by fear to seek out health care methods I thought unsafe. I knew, however, that *having* the book and the indicated remedy on hand had made all the difference that night. It was clear that I—and other parents who wanted to treat their children's illnesses by natural methods—would need a lot of tested information to succeed at this and feel secure.

Many of my patients and friends with children, tired of penicillin and child care books that constantly urged them to "see a physician," had expressed their desire for a book like this. I had always meant to collect the information and—now that I knew how it felt to *be* the worried, distracted, sleepless parent—I undertook the project with more vehemence. I went to conferences and seminars, discussed the subject with other doctors, read cases, pored over books, advised willing patients on self-care measures, and collected a wealth of remedies that parents could use effectively with safety and confidence.

Many of the treatments suggested can work together to help a child overcome disease, but often (especially with homeopathic remedies) the use of one will be sufficient. Children all have their tastes and idiosyncrasies: some love herb teas and others hate them; some enjoy massage and acupressure while others jump out of their skins; some will proudly swallow vitamins and some gag or spit them out. Parents should sanely consider the various therapies listed, and choose the approach that suits their child best. Although intended for parents, this book will also be useful to anyone closely involved in the lives of children: grandparents, teachers, daycare workers, doctors, nurses, dentists, and open-minded health practitioners of all persuasions, who may also effectively use these treatments on themselves.

Part One addresses the use of common natural health care methods: Homeopathy, Nutrition, Herbal Medicine, and Acupressure. While many parents have had experience with some or all of these techniques, others may want to study the background information before beginning to use them. Appendices in the back of the book provide more detail and specific information.

Part Two contains a section on Emergencies, sections on Poisoning and Shock, and a section on Drugs and Modern Medical Procedures, which cites some dangerous side effects of treatments often prescribed by conventional medical doctors. Following these is a section on Immunizations, in which the theory behind the use of vaccines for disease-prevention, the very real risks of this practice, the rights of children and parents in regard to immunization, and some possible alternatives are discussed.

Part Three, the main body of the book, consists of alphabetically arranged sections that deal with particular illnesses or health concerns that arise in children's lives. Each of these sections includes:

- A definition and short explanation of what is going on in a child's body when the condition occurs; its causes, signs, and symptoms; guidance in determining its severity, and when it is best to seek a physician's help.
- Information about the accepted or standard medical procedures related to the condition: what types of examination and treatment might be employed by an allopathically-oriented doctor, and questions or problems that might arise with that approach.
- Natural treatments or methods of prevention that have been found to be helpful to children with that condition, including (when applicable) foods and nutritional supplements, herbs, homeopathic remedies, acupressure points, and other practical measures including relaxation exercises, prevention tips, and miscellaneous treatments to increase a child's comfort.

Part Four contains appendices with more detailed information on homeopathic remedies, nutrition, herbs, and acupressure, and ends with a list of books that may help increase understanding of health care methods described in the text.

Certain children's maladies are part of life and almost unavoidable. There are others, however, that occur rarely or are very mild if the child's habits are healthy. Nutritious food, amusing exercise, pure water, clean air, and a relaxed and interesting environment can help keep a child's system strong and resilient. Foods that are refined and processed (especially sugar), artificial flavorings, colorings and sweeteners, chemical additives, pollution, radiation, excessive exposure to television or computers, suppressive medical treatments, drug and alcohol use, and unhappy family and school situations can work against a child's health.

Problems with drugs and alcohol, abuse and violence, and sexually transmitted diseases are serious concerns that go beyond the scope of a natural health care book. Counselors or health care specialists whose attitudes are balanced and nonthreatening can often help a troubled child. Developmental defects, heart problems, hormone imbalance, and rare or very serious illnesses are also not discussed here at length; such conditions need a doctor's close attention, although natural therapies used as adjuncts to a physician's treatment may strengthen the child and facilitate other medical care.

While one of the goals of this book is to help parents become more self-sufficient and confident in taking care of a child who is ill, its information is not intended to take the place of a doctor's care at any time that it is truly warranted. If a child is very uncomfortable, behaves abnormally, or fails to respond to natural treatments within a reasonable length of time, a physician's help should be sought.

It is best to find a physician you can trust and call on, *before* your child gets ill. A good pediatrician can be hard to find, so you may have to do some exploring. Ask other parents for names of physicians they like and would recommend. Ask other types of healers in your area (chiropractors, naturopaths, nutritionists, and acupuncturists) for names of medical doctors with whom they can work without conflict. Call a number of offices and ask about the doctors' attitudes toward natural treatments; try to arrange a time to talk with the doctors themselves. This may eliminate the need to go to an emergency room and receive possibly dangerous treatment from doctors who do not know your child.

Look for a doctor who respects the body's healing tendencies and is not too quick to reach for the drug prescription pad. Many physicians reject the validity of natural therapies merely because these were not included in their training; look for a doctor who willingly answers questions and does not feel threatened by subjects on which he or she is not well-informed. Bring up some of the points discussed in various sections of this book: How will the doctor feel if you choose to save invasive measures such as drugs and X rays for emergency situations? If your child had to be hospitalized with a serious infection, would the doctor be willing to give high doses of intravenous vitamins at your request? If you chose to use natural therapies to treat your children's minor illnesses, would the doctor support this, and still be willing to help if the need for drastic treatment arose? Keep looking until you find a physician your child likes, who has good rapport with both of you, and an attitude that will work with your own.

Most of all, learn as much as you can to help you make wise decisions and tend to your children's health care needs with confidence. Besides being inexpensive and convenient to use, natural treatments really work, and using them can make your family's life more balanced, pleasant, and comfortable.

HOMEOPATHY

Homeopathy is a very effective and interesting system of healing that has been used to treat illness and injury for nearly two hundred years. It is widely accepted in Europe and India and is becoming increasingly popular in the United States and Latin America. Near the turn of the century, nearly one-quarter of all American doctors identified themselves as homeopaths. Political pressures from the American Medical Association leading to financial and licensure limitations subsequently made it difficult for doctors to practice homeopathic medicine, and the rate of professional use declined. Despite such pressures, there have always been doctors persistently studying and practicing homeopathy—and in recent years, as patients have turned to non-invasive medicine—their numbers have grown larger.

Homeopathic medicine differs from allopathic medicine (the standard approach of modern medical doctors) in important ways. Allopathic physicians regard symptoms as manifestations of disease and often work to oppose or suppress them. An M.D. might, for example, prescribe aspirin to reduce a fever, a drug to relax a muscle spasm, or cortisone to reduce inflammation of joints or skin. A homeopath, in contrast, considers symptoms evidence that the body's internal defenses against disease are working. On the basis of specific symptoms, a homeopathic remedy is chosen to bolster the body's healing powers and eventually help restore its balanced function. Homeopathic medicine is holistic in approach, in keeping with the belief that all parts of a human being—body, mind, and emotions—are interdependent. Homeopathy as a science is backed by a great body of literature based on observation and clinical experience.

The term *homeopathy* comes from the Greek words *homoios* (similar) and *pathos* (suffering or disease). Homeopathic treatment is based on the principle, *Similia similibus curentur:* "Let like be cured by like." The theory behind the homeopathic system is that each of the remedy substances, if taken in crude form or excess, can *cause* in healthy persons a particular set or complex of symptoms. When a person becomes ill, a remedy is chosen by observing the symptoms carefully and selecting the substance whose remedy picture most closely matches the state that person is experiencing.

For example, the remedy *Apis mellifica* is made from the venom and body of the honeybee. Most of us have been stung by bees and know the typical symptoms: painful stinging, burning sensation, heat and inflammation relieved by cold applications, puffy pink swelling, extreme tenderness to touch, emotional upset or irritability. *Apis mellifica,* when prepared as a homeopathic remedy, is used for conditions such as allergy, sore throat, eye inflammations, measles, chicken pox, hives, and insect bites, which are characterized by stinging, burning, hot, pink, puffy swelling, are tender to touch and relieved by cold applications, and make the person upset or irritable. Another example is *Allium cepa,* made from red onion. The symptoms caused by raw onions—red, teary eyes and runny noses—when encountered in conditions such as colds or allergies are frequently cured by *Allium cepa* prepared as a homeopathic remedy.

In many situations, choosing the proper remedy can be this simple. At other times more study, observation, and detective work are needed. This work is worth the effort. As an alternative therapy, homeopathy is gratifying: correctly chosen, the remedies really work! Many parents who at one time dutifully gave their children toxic chemicals as medications, often against their instinctive suspicion that such drugs were harmful, have learned to safely treat their children's headaches, flus, or ear infections with homeopathic remedies. They now have the confidence to handle the family's nonemergency illnesses themselves—to help, without doing harm.

Homeopathic remedies are made from hundreds of different single substances of mineral, plant, and animal origin, prepared in such a way that they are completely nontoxic. Unlike allopathic drugs, which often interfere with natural body processes in order to suppress or alter symptoms, homeopathic remedies gently stimulate and organize a person's internal disease-fighting powers and help the body regain its strength and health.

Homeopathic remedies are always given in *potentized* form.

Potentization is a special method of preparing a medicinal substance by putting it through a series of dilutions and succussions. (Succussion is a vigorous shaking action.) This process allows the curative force of a substance to operate, while removing any possibility of chemical toxicity. Even though substances prepared for remedies may be diluted tens, hundreds, or thousands of times, it has been found that they become, with each dilution and succussion, more "potent." That is, the higher the potency, the more capable the remedy seems to be of touching the patient on deep internal levels and helping the body's defenses effect an efficient cure.

An important distinction between homeopathic and allopathic medicine is that homeopathic remedies are chosen to match a person's specific symptoms, rather than to treat a named disease or diagnosis. For instance, if a child is ill, in order to select a remedy the parent must first take careful note of the symptoms: Which are the most distinct or troublesome? What sensations (such as burning, trembling, numbness, itching, cramping) accompany them? What influences (heat, cold, rest, motion, position, touch, eating, drinking) seem to make them better or worse? The child's appearance, emotions, and mental state may also be factors in finding the remedy.

Imagine that two children in one family are feeling sick. The sister is nauseous, anxious, and hates the smell of food but constantly wants to sip hot tea; she is chilly and wants a pile of blankets on her bed, but gets up at intervals to pace the room. Her brother has griping stomach pains, fever, and headache; he takes long cold drinks, doesn't answer questions, and wants to lie still and be left alone. These children both have "the flu," but different homeopathic remedies would be prescribed for them.

When choosing a remedy, study the child's condition carefully. Read all of the remedy indications in the appropriate section(s) of this book. If the child exhibits symptoms of more than one condition (for instance, both headache and stomachache), consider all the listed information and take time to select the *single remedy* that fits the picture best. If a perfect match is hard to find, choose the remedy that best matches the most intense or unusual symptoms and the child's general state—mood, temperature, and appetite. This careful consideration will save trouble later. Doubting your prescription may make you go on to other remedies too quickly, and disrupt the work of the first before it has had a chance to show its good effect.

One important point to remember when choosing remedies for children is to try to get them to use their own words to describe how they feel. "Does anything in your body bother you?" is a better question "Does your head hurt?" "How does your tummy feel?" is better than "Does your tummy burn?" "What would you like to eat or drink?" is better than "How about cold orange juice?" Some children (especially small ones) may try to give you the answer they think you're after—which won't help you find the remedy to make them well.

Once the single best remedy has been chosen, *one dose* of a lower potency—6X, 6C, 12X, 12C, 30X, or 30C—should be given (these numbers and letters refer to the dilution level). One dose is usually one tablet, one larger pellet, several smaller pellets, or several drops, depending upon which form of the remedy is used. Observe the child's response for an hour or more. If the remedy given was the correct one, the child will gradually experience relief of symptoms.

If the remedy appears to be working and the child's symptoms are easing, however slowly, *do not repeat* the remedy unless improvement stops. If symptoms return or the child's condition seems to have leveled off and is not improving further, the remedy may be given again. How long to wait at this point is partly based on common sense: a throbbing headache will require more prompt attention than a bout of constipation or a week-old ankle sprain.

If a child has a cold or flu that might normally last a week, a well-selected remedy may ease a great deal of discomfort and shorten the length of the illness by several days. Usually a repetition of a remedy that has worked initially, then lagged, will cause improvement to resume. If, however, the repeated dose seems to have brought no response within an hour or two, you should consider the child's present symptoms (including emotional ones) and see if another remedy fits them. Remember, you will help your child more if you are not impatient or hasty to repeat or change the remedy. Homeopathic remedies do wonderful things, and sometimes results are almost instantaneous, but don't expect magic.

A person cannot be poisoned by an overdose of homeopathic remedies: an entire bottle of tablets could be swallowed with no ill effect. But the power of these remedies should not be taken lightly. Because they work on an energy level, repeated doses of incorrectly chosen remedies, or even correct ones repeated much too frequently, may confuse the symptom picture and interrupt the curative effect.

In order to be sure that the remedy itself is not inactivated, it is important to observe the following precautions.

· Have the child take the remedy at least fifteen minutes after eating or drinking anything. Then wait at least fifteen minutes more before any food or drink or anything else (such as gum, cough drops, or toothpaste) goes into the mouth.

· When opening the remedy vial, make sure there are no strong smells (such as perfume, camphor, paint fumes, mothballs, aromatic herbs) in the room, as these may denature a remedy.

· Try not to touch the actual remedy. Pellets or tablets may be tapped into the vial cap or onto a clean slip of paper and tipped directly onto or under the child's tongue to dissolve. They should not be swallowed or chewed. The pellets and tablets will taste slightly sweet from their base of mild milk sugar.

· Take care during homeopathic treatment to avoid all antidoting influences—substances that deactivate remedies, such as camphor, coffee, and allopathic drugs, unless, as in the case of insulin or steroid drugs, the child has become dependent on them. Analgesic ointments, herbal salves, lip balms, and cough drops often contain camphor. Coffee is sometimes an ingredient of candies, desserts, ice cream, or baked goods. Often these aren't a problem, but you can't be sure, so caution is better. Even decaffeinated coffee has been known to antidote remedies.

Homeopathic remedies can be used along with antibiotics or allopathic drugs if, in some very serious condition, these are truly needed; more frequent repetitions will usually have to be made, and the remedies may not have the chance to work as well, but they still may help the person recover more quickly.

Most remedies can be easily obtained through the mail from homeopathic pharmacies, some of which are listed in the Appendix. Many of these pharmacies sell home first-aid kits, which can include up to fifty remedies. In a number of cities, natural food stores or shops that specialize in herbs and vitamins also carry the more common remedies. Families should either purchase a remedy kit or assemble their own kit by buying remedies separately. Such kits are a good investment: having the common remedies on hand may help to relieve discomfort, shorten illnesses, and often obviate the need for expensive and toxic medications.

Some stores also offer combination remedies labeled for specific disorders, such as headache, bedwetting and indigestion. Although combination remedies are at times effective, the use of single remedies is usually preferable. For one thing, the use of single remedies removes confusion. If a combination remedy cures the symptoms, which of the six or eight included remedies is the one that acted? If the combination doesn't work, it is also puzzling. Was the needed remedy *not* included in the mixture, or have the various remedies confused the case or canceled one another out?

Another source of possible confusion: The Food and Drug Administration (FDA) is now requiring homeopathic pharmacies to label remedies with "therapeutic indications." Since correct prescribing of the remedies is based on qualities and characteristic symptoms in each remedy picture, and since each of the remedies may work, *when indicated,* for a wide variety of health conditions, this form of compulsory labeling is misleading and limiting. A father, for instance, having studied this book and chosen *Chamomilla* for his daughter's fever and stabbing ear pain, would be puzzled to see the bottle labeled "for irritability and sleeplessness." A mother could rush for *Cantharis* to soothe her son's burned fingers, only to find it labeled for "urinary tract infections." It is sad to think that labeling restrictions supposedly enforced to protect consumers but based, in this case, on ignorance of homeopathic science, may be dissuading people from easing illness and pain with these safe, effective medicines.

The homeopathic remedies mentioned in this book are, for the most part, to be used in acute care of fairly ordinary health conditions. If a person has a very serious disease or deep-seated problem, it is best to seek "classical" constitutional treatment from a qualified homeopathic prescriber, and, if needed, emergency allopathic help. In other situations, however, the amateur student of homeopathy will find that knowing and using these remedies will bring the family a lot of cheer and confidence.

To gain the maximum benefits from homeopathy, I recommend that you read other books on the subject, some of which I've listed in Recommended Reading. Also, please see the first Appendix in the back of this book for a list of homeopathic remedies and pharmacies.

Fresh fruits and vegetables, edible seeds, whole grains, and high-quality protein will make up a nourishing diet for a child for not much more than the cost of high-fat, empty-calorie processed food. It isn't difficult to provide a balanced, healthful diet for a child, yet the eating habits of our culture do not exactly encourage this. Even if parents give their children good food, the children don't always eat it. Many youngsters have vehement preferences for junk food, candy, and desserts. A sweet tooth is actually part of the natural human palate: foods rich in natural vitamin C, such as fruits and berries, are sweet; but most sweets in our diet today are robbed by refinement of vitamins and minerals and, being far too concentrated, work against the body's health. Fruit still satisfies this yen for sweets, however, so have fruit on hand to offer your child.

Fortunately during the last few years a number of healthy versions of popular snacks and other foods have been developed: cereals, pretzels, crackers, chips, cheese puffs, cookies, and breads that are chemical-free and made of whole grains. Cookies, candy, cakes, and ice cream sweetened with fruit or honey can be found in natural food stores. Goat's-milk products and rice- or soy-based versions of dairy foods are being provided in tastier forms. Vegetables, fruits, beans, and grains grown organically and without pesticides, as well as poultry and meats (even hot dogs) produced without antibiotics, hormones, or chemicals, can be bought in many places. Those who can afford to buy as many foods as possible from organic farms and smaller nutrition-minded companies can assure themselves that the better nutrition is worth the money. The more support the organic farmers and natural food producers receive from consumers, the wider their sales will be and the sooner their prices will become competitive.

VITAMIN AND MINERAL SUPPLEMENTS

As knowledge of the actual workings of nutrients in the body has developed, it has become more clear that to stay truly healthy certain individuals (possibly all of us) need more nutrients than a normal diet provides. Supplements of vitamins and minerals used in moderation seem to encourage better health in many people. The Recommended Daily Allowance (RDA) of nutrients reflect amounts that are likely only to prevent the blatant symptoms of deficiency. Many stresses in the modern world, however, make our bodies require more nutrients than they would if we had a simpler, more natural way of life: toxic chemicals, radiation, and other stresses deplete our bodies of nutrients.

Much of our food is grown on depleted soil and fertilized with chemicals to encourage crops that appear big and healthy without being very nutritious. Pesticides are used to ensure that the plants appear robust, but toxic residues remain in the foods we eat. Animals, poultry, and even fish are often raised in unnatural, miserable conditions with emphasis placed on appearance, not nutrition. Food is heavily processed: refining flours, grains, and sugar takes away more vital nutrients than are later replaced by "enrichment." Colorings, dyes, waxes, bleaches, and other food cosmetics are used to cover evidence that fruits and vegetables have been forced to a certain size and picked before ripe, that grains and flours are not always really fresh. Air and water are no longer pure. Hardly an unpolluted spot remains in the world; wastes from industry, transportation, and power production constantly poison living things and alter nature. Both medical and nonmedical drugs, tobacco, alcohol, job and school pressures, crowding, nervous tension, and psychological stress all increase people's needs for nutrients. Aware of this information, many people take nutritional supplements and give them to their children.

This is not to say that supplements should be used without restraint. Gross overuse of supplements can be harmful in certain cases, and tremendously expensive. Still, a basic multivitamin, multimineral supplement can fill the gaps that remain from a less than perfect diet and help the body deal with stress and abnormal substances. During illness and many health conditions, extra amounts of certain nutrients can be helpful. Nutrients used to help the body overcome illness are not being used as drugs; drugs are abnormal substances that chemically alter body processes and change the symptoms of illness. In contrast, vitamins and minerals are recognized by the body as part of food.

Natural vs. synthetic is a question that arises when looking for supplements. Since the body recognizes vitamins as necessary elements, it makes sense to use the natural forms, from which the synthetic forms often differ slightly. In the case of vitamins A and D especially this is important, as the natural and artificial forms appear to be used in different ways by the body. Also, many trace minerals and nutritive elements act as synergists (or helpers) to vitamins; these are often found together with their partners in natural foods. If these synergists are not included in supplements, and vitamins are supplied from synthetic sources, the necessary elements and combinations may not be present to do their work.

Many "natural" vitamins are actually made up of small amounts from a food source augmented with larger doses of the synthetic form. In many cases this is unavoidable; for instance, deriving large amounts of B vitamins from food alone would make the supplements so bulky and expensive that no one would use them. As is the case with many products of industry, it is hard to be sure of what you're getting when buying supplements. Price does not always relate to quality. The cheapest brands, or those mass-produced by drug or oil companies, may not provide good nutrition. The most expensive ones, however, are not necessarily better than those in the middle price range. Consulting with nutritionists and reading health care literature may help you decide which supplements to choose.

Look for children's chewable multivitamin and mineral tablets that are free of sugar, artificial flavors, sweeteners, and colorings, and that also taste good. A child who swallows pills without discomfort can be given any supplement in a dose that suits his age and size. If chewing or swallowing pills isn't feasible, tablets may be crushed to powder, or capsules opened and the contents mixed with small amounts of foods like applesauce or yogurt. A "chaser" of something tasty afterward may help the dose go down. Take care to give all nutrients in moderation, especially those for which the infant's and children's doses are not established, keeping in mind the child's age and size.

Please see Appendix for a listing of recommended dosages of supplements for children, as well as foods in which these nutrients can be found.

HERBAL MEDICINE

Herbs have been used as medicine throughout recorded history; in fact, it is easy to imagine that their inclusion in the natural world is for this purpose. Hundreds of plants have beneficial and medicinal effects on the human body, just as many other plants are used as foods. Sophisticated and effective approaches to healing, such as Chinese medicine and Ayurveda, include a deep understanding of herbs and specific combinations of them. Many medical drugs in use today have been developed on the basis of information derived from the physiological effects of herbs. Herbs in their natural form, however, are more balanced in action and safer than drugs.

Before using herbs, you need to know which ones are safe, in what amounts, and which ones have dangerous effects. Just as we have learned to eat tomatoes but not their relative, deadly night-shade, and to recognize the carrot as food but not the poison camas-root, we can easily learn to choose the medicinal herbs that will soothe and make us well, not kill us. There is, however, a borderland: some herbs are very useful medicines, yet their doses must be closely monitored. Dangerous or complicated herbs should be left in the hands of expert herbalists and naturopathic doctors; people use them in their homes with good results, but this should never be tried without clear knowledge of their properties and dosages. Only nontoxic, very safe uses of herbs are included in this book. Still, it is wise to monitor your child's reaction carefully.

In the following sections are lists of herbs that may be used as teas to help children recover from illness. Giving them singly rather than several in combination will help you see your child's response to individual herbs. Honey and lemon may be added to suit your child's palate and help the herbal teas go down. Teas may be cooled and mixed with strong-tasting fruit juice (black cherry or grape, for instance) or given in gulps or spoonfuls with a favorite juice as a "chaser," quickly followed by a teaspoon of honey, some raisins, or something else tasty.

Introduce new herbs in moderation: any food, chemical, natural, or artificial substance can be an allergen or disagree with someone who is sensitive. If symptoms such as headache, skin rash, stomachache, or diarrhea occur within an hour or so of taking any herb, do not continue giving it; choose some other treatment for that child.

Most of the herbs listed in this book can be purchased in herb shops or natural food stores. Some are grown in gardens or found in fields or woodlands. If you are using herbs from fields or woods, be absolutely sure of their identity; consult an herbalist or check with an herb book (see the Appendix of Recommended Reading). Most herbs are sold dried, either loose or in teabags, while some are used in fresh form, especially those that are also foods or seasonings. To retain their potency, herbs should be placed in clean, airtight containers and stored in a dark, cool, dry place.

Herbs can be taken in many ways—oils, tinctures, powders, poultices—but the most common usage recommended in this book is in teas. To make herbal tea, steep or simmer one to two teaspoonfuls of herb in one cup of boiling water for five to ten minutes. (For larger amounts or stronger infusions, vary proportions accordingly.) Use a strainer to separate the bits of plant from the liquid, and cool the tea to a comfortable temperature for drinking. Freshly made teas are most reliable, though many will keep refrigerated for a day or two. Herbal teas can also be used as a skin-wash or as an infusion added to baths.

Herbal oils are occasionally recommended in the text; they can be useful as insect repellents or as applications for skin eruptions. They are usually purchased premade, but you can make your own by covering the fresh herb with olive oil in a clean jar or bottle and letting it stand for two to three weeks.

Herbal powders for gargles and external applications may be made by grinding the dried root, herb, or seeds in a clean coffee grinder or grain-mill.

Tinctures can be made by combining an ounce of herb with four to eight ounces of alcohol (brandy or vodka) and letting the mixture stand for two to three weeks, shaking once or twice a day.

Poultices are usually made by crushing or stewing fresh plants, or mixing dry herbs with warm water, and placing them directly on the skin. This may be messy and some herbs, like comfrey, are prickly. It may be more convenient to wrap the herbs in a thin, clean, dampened cloth.

The Glossary of Herbs in the Appendices gives a brief description of herbs suggested for use in the various sections of this book.

ACUPRESSURE

The stimulation of specific points on the body by means of finger pressure, (often referred to as acupressure), reflexology, and specific massage have been part of many healing systems and cultures for thousands of years. These techniques are based on the theory that the body contains energy (bioenergy, or in the Chinese tradition, *ch'i*), considered to be the essence of life which, ideally, runs smoothly and harmoniously throughout a healthy body. Various influences—stress or nutritional deficiencies, for example—may create an internal imbalance and interrupt the flow of bioenergy, contributing to disease. Acupressure works by breaking these energy blocks through fingertip stimulation of specific points, balancing the flow of *ch'i* through the meridians, and stimulating the body's ability to heal itself.

The acupressure and reflex points mentioned in this book are only a few among thousands that are part of healing systems such as acupuncture, shiatsu, polarity, and zone therapy. They have been chosen because they are effective for many common conditions, and because the points are easy to find and treat on children, who often find comfort from the process.

To use acupressure on your child, press or rub each indicated point for a minute or so. Apply deep but never hard or painful pressure on the points. The child may feel tenderness or increased sensitivity at the point of stimulation; this is a sign that you've found the right spot. All points that are not on the midline should be treated on both sides of the body. Points should be worked once a day, or more often if necessary, as long as symptoms are present.

Things to remember when using acupressure:
- Be sure the child is in a comfortable position and can relax during treatment.
- Be sure the room, and your hands, are warm enough for the child's comfort.
- Make sure your hands are clean and your fingernails trimmed before rubbing points on the child's skin.

- Do not use acupressure on a child who has a very full stomach or who has taken medications within the last hour or so, as these can interfere with the flow of energy and inhibit the treatment's effects.
- To avoid the possibility of damage, do not use acupressure points in areas of injury, scarring, or infection.
- If working a point appears to aggravate symptoms, do not continue using it.

The treatment's effectiveness can enhanced if you imagine healing energy moving from your hands to the child. Older children can be encouraged to stimulate their own acupressure points.

The Appendix on Acupressure lists the traditional acupuncture points suggested for treatment throughout this book, along with illustrated diagrams showing the exact body location of those points. Additional areas for specific massage are also described in various sections.

PART 2
MEDICAL AWARENESS

EMERGENCIES

The difference between life and death, relief and disaster, may lie in the way you handle an emergency. It is important that you know what to do in case of emergency and act immediately rather than letting panic cloud your judgment or wasting precious time.

You should know (and have written down for visitors or baby-sitters) the quickest route to the nearest hospital and the telephone numbers of the closest fire department or rescue squad. (For most of us, this number is 911.) You should also have readily available the numbers for a poison control center, the nearest emergency room, and neighbors whom you can call for help. Make sure your child knows how to dial 911 and how to give clear directions to your home.

FIRST-AID KIT

A kit containing clean bandages, gauze, and absorbent cotton in unopened sterile packages, paper tissues, antiseptic, tweezers, and scissors should be kept in a clean, dry metal or plastic container and stored in a convenient place. Some families have two kits: one for home and one kept in the car for use while traveling. Natural items that should be included are: tinctures of calendula, hypericum, and ledum for use as antiseptics for cuts, infections, and puncture wounds; aloe vera gel and vitamin E oil for burns; a dropper-bottle of Rescue Remedy, the Bach Flower remedy for shock and serious injury; and the homeopathic remedies *Arnica* for bruising and shock; *Apis mellifica* and *Carbolicum acidum* for dangerous swelling from bites or stings, and allergic shock; *Cantharis* for burns; *Hypericum* for injuries to nerves; and *Ledum* for puncture wounds. A larger home remedy kit with twenty to fifty other homeopathic remedies may also come in handy.

Bach Flower Remedies and homeopathic remedies can be bought in some herb shops or natural food stores, or can be ordered through the mail. For a list of homeopathic pharmacies, see the first Appendix at the back of this book.

RESUSCITATION

Call the local fire department or hospital and inquire whether a CPR course is offered in your area. Take the course and have your children take it too, if possible.

Remember the sequence ABC—Airway, Breathing, Circulation if breathing or heartbeat has stopped.

A. Airway
1. Pull the tongue forward; quickly clear any mucus or foreign matter from the mouth and throat.
2. Have the child lying on his back; tilt his head back and pull his jaw forward.

B. Breathing
3. Pinch his nose so the nostrils stay closed, and cover his mouth with yours. (For a baby or very small child, cover mouth and nose with your mouth.)
4. Blow air in with enough force to make his chest visibly rise; give one breath every three to four seconds. (For a tiny baby, blow with gentle puffs, about once every two seconds.)

C. Circulation
5. If the heart has stopped beating, place the heel of your hand against the lower half of the breastbone (not the very tip) and push down firmly enough to temporarily depress it about an inch; do this about once per second. A good pattern is five breaths, five compressions; five breaths, five compressions, etc.
6. Keep this up for an hour or more, or until breathing starts again; while you are doing this, have someone else go for help. The fire department or rescue squad can usually bring help quickly and provide oxygen.

Note. Touch a drop of Rescue Remedy or homeopathic *Arnica* to the inner lining of the cheek; repeat this every few minutes, while continuing CPR, until you see a response.

CHOKING

If you can't reach in and pull out the obstruction, hold the child head-down across your arm or lap and give sharp pats between the shoulder blades until the object is coughed out.

If for some reason the child cannot be held upside down, perform the *Heimlich maneuver.* With the child upright, stand behind her, put the flat of your hand between her navel and rib cage, and give a quick "bear hug" upwards.

This may also be done with the child lying on her back. Kneeling beside her, press the heel of your hand between rib cage and navel and give several quick upward pushes. If the child is very small, use two flat fingertips instead of the heel of the hand.

If these moves do not help, get professional help as quickly as possible.

PREVENTION. Do not let small children play with toys that have tiny parts that come off. Up to the age of three or four these always end up in the mouth. Do not let babies chew on styrofoam. Bits may come off and be inhaled, and the fumes may be toxic. Remind children (and adults) not to run, jump, or actively play with gum or other objects in their mouths.

Do not give fruit with seeds, popcorn, nuts, sunflower seeds, gum, hard candy, or any food that comes apart in pieces to children under four unless you are there every second, watching. Teach children of all ages to chew their food completely before they swallow. Meat, hot dogs, grapes, sticky candy, dried fruits, and other foods can get stuck and block the windpipe.

ELECTRIC SHOCK

If the child is stuck to the source of current, do not pull her away with your hands—you also will become part of the circuit. Separate her from it by means of an object made of wood, (such as a broom handle), cloth (loop a dry towel or shirt around and pull her away), rubber, plastic, or some other nonconductor. Use nothing wet or made of metal. If the child is in shock or has stopped breathing, immediately begin emergency procedures (see RESUSCITATION above; see also BURNS in Part Three).

DROWNING

If a child is underwater, unconscious, get her out immediately. Give her mouth-to-mouth resuscitation immediately, even before reaching the water's edge, as seconds sometimes make the difference between life and death. If air will not enter her lungs which may mean they are full of water, put her head lower than her feet, tilt her on her side, and press against her abdomen between rib cage and navel with a sharp upward thrust. After some water has come out, resume resuscitation immediately.

The homeopathic remedy *Antimonium tartaricum* has been known to help drowning victims. After administering mouth-to-mouth breathing, crush the tablets or pellets into powder or dissolve them in a little water and touch the remedy to the inner lining of the child's cheek. Repeat this every few minutes until she shows improvement.

BLEEDING

If bleeding is serious and hard to control, raise the bleeding part as high as possible, then press firmly directly against the wound with a clean cloth, the cleanest garment you can find, or your hand or arm. If you can locate a bone, push the cut blood vessel against that, on the side of the wound closest to the heart, so that the blood will not continue to be pumped out and will have a chance to form a clot. Send someone for help, and keep pressing—for hours if necessary, until the bleeding stops. (See also BLEEDING in Part Three.)

TRAUMATIC INJURY or FRACTURE

Do not move a seriously injured person, especially if there is any possibility of fracture of the skull, neck, spine, or ribs. Keep the person calm and treat for shock if necessary. (See SHOCK below.) Call 911 immediately.

CHILLING and HYPOTHERMIA

Chilling can occur from exposure to wintry weather, wind, wearing wet clothes, being in an unheated house, or being unable to maintain body temperature because of fatigue, hunger, inactivity, or inefficient metabolism.

The method of treatment depends on how cold the child is. If his skin feels as though it has no warmth in it—not just the hands and feet, but the chest and other areas under the clothes—it may be that his body is temporarily incapable of raising the body heat. In such a case, adding layers of bedding or clothing might actually seal in the cold. A better approach would be to first warm the child slowly—by bringing him into a warmer room, giving him warm drinks to sip, or having him snuggle up against a warm person or dog. Once the child's body is bringing up its own heat, extra coverings will help it along. If the child is severely chilled (hypothermic), professional help may be needed. Warm bathing is not recommended in such a case, as it may cause the cold blood in the extremities to move toward the more vital areas of the body.

Sometimes a newborn or very small infant becomes chilled while in deep sleep; this happens because the warming mechanism inside her body hasn't had much practice yet. Usually a baby will breathe rapidly and cry when she's cold, but if she has become still and limp, difficult to rouse, uninterested in nursing, with skin very cold to the touch (sometimes with feet and hands that look bright pink and swollen), this can be an emergency. Hold her close to your own body for warmth, and keep her in a warm room (or car), away from exposure to damp or cold air. Expert help should be sought immediately, while attempts are made to warm the baby—gently, but quickly. (For chills, see FEVER in Part Three.)

ANAPHYLACTIC SHOCK

This type of shock is caused by a life-threatening allergic reaction. If adrenaline is available, inject it immediately (one-quarter milliliter for children). Or give the homeopathic remedy *Apis* in the highest potency available. If it does not act, try *Carbolicum acidum.* Get medical help as quickly as possible. (See also SHOCK below and ALLERGIES in Part Three.)

SHOCK

Shock is a condition in which the blood flow to vital organs is deranged, as a reaction to an injury, dehydration, poisoning, a drug or allergen, severe infection, or other trauma.

A child experiencing shock may seem dizzy, confused, less alert than usual; her skin may be pale and cold; her earlobes, lips, and fingernails may look blue; her heartbeat may be fast and weak; her mouth dry and breathing shallow. She may feel thirsty, but should not be given fluids, in case she loses consciousness and inhales the liquid.

These symptoms are caused when the brain and vital organs are deprived of the circulation they need to function correctly. Circulation may be deranged by severe bleeding, or by the nervous system's inefficient reaction to trauma, causing the blood to pool in less vital areas.

Some treatment for shock by a physician will be the same as home care: the person must be kept warm, and circulation to the brain encouraged. Any bleeding will be controlled and obstruction of breathing corrected. If necessary the child will be given oxygen. Extra fluids are often given by IV, and drugs may be given to control blood pressure.

If a child goes into shock, call 911 or otherwise seek emergency care. While help is on the way, follow the practical measures listed below.

PRACTICAL MEASURES. Shock should be treated right away. Even if its cause is not serious, the condition of shock itself can be dangerous, even life-threatening. If shock is due to heavy bleeding, dehydration, or another known cause, give first aid. (See BLEEDING above and in Part Three, and DEHYDRATION in Part Three.) If a child is in shock for *any* reason, summon help or take her to an emergency room right away.

While waiting or going for help, have the child lie down in

the *Recovery position*: on her tummy with her head turned to one side, with the leg and arm on that side drawn up at right angles. This will help prevent suffocation from saliva or vomit. Loosen any tight clothing that might restrict breathing. Put pillows or rolled-up clothes under her hips and legs so her head will be lower than the rest of her body, which helps more blood reach the brain. She should be covered with blankets and kept warm. Keep her company and comfort her, trying to reduce her apprehension, as fear can increase the shock reaction. Do not give anything by mouth except for homeopathic remedies, which, in powder or droplet form should be touched to the mucous membrane on the inside of the cheek.

Rescue Remedy, a combination of Bach Flower Remedies, or the single remedy Rock Rose, may be give every five minutes until improvement is seen.

HOMEOPATHIC REMEDIES.
> *Arnica montana*—the main remedy given for shock, especially if the shock has been caused by physical injury.
> *Apis mellifica*—for anaphylactic, allergic shock caused by a bee-sting or a drug reaction; if *Apis* does not work, use *Carbolicum acidum*. (See ALLERGIES in Part Three.)
> *Carbo vegetabilis*—child is very cold (though head may be hot); pale; weak pulse; desperate for air.
> *Phosphorus*—for extreme loss of blood.

ACUPRESSURE AND MASSAGE.
- GV 26: A point in the middle of the groove above the upper lip (press with thumbnail).
- Pinch the end of the middle fingers on both sides of the nailbed.
- Massage the arches of the feet and hands, and briskly wiggle the toes, wrists, and fingers; this can help the nervous system and adrenal glands restore circulation.

POISONING

One of the ways that babies and small children explore the world is by putting things in their mouths. Many older children are adventurous and like to experiment: they may grasp the *concept* of poisoning, but it may be hard for them to understand its real results and dangers. Some children may seem very sedate or cautious and never take risks—then suddenly, on a whim, take a sip from the gas can or eat the deodorant.

Children can be accidentally or inadvertently poisoned in other ways than by swallowing the wrong thing. Many common household chemicals, such as bug sprays, cosmetics, lighter fluid, typist's correction fluid, cleaning products, polishes, solvents, wood preservatives, paints, and varnishes, send dangerous fumes into the air and into the family's lungs. Some toxic substances are absorbed through the skin into the bloodstream. Because the immediate symptoms of such poisoning are often slight (a headache or temporary irritability) many people do not realize that the liver, brain, and other tissues of the body may be receiving permanent damage from such exposure, and the risk of immune system weakness or cancer may be increased.

Signs of poisoning may include stomach pains, diarrhea, nausea, vomiting, rapid deep breathing, a flushed or hot face, burning mouth, unusual sleepiness, convulsions, and unconsciousness. If a child has been exposed to any poison and is in pain, disoriented, or unconscious, go to an emergency room or get expert help immediately.

PRACTICAL MEASURES. The best way to avoid poisoning is to keep everything that is unsafe for a child out of reach and out of sight. Your poison control center can send you a list of common poisonous substances and the proper course to follow if they are swallowed. Remember that all medications, alcoholic beverages, vitamin supplements, and even some spices can be poisonous if large amounts are swallowed. Know which plants in your house, yard, or woods are poisonous. Surfaces in old houses, of old furniture, or other objects may be coated with paint containing lead. Imported objects or ceramics may also have lead-containing paints or glazes. Keep all nonfood substances in the house, garage, or outbuildings on high shelves or in locked cupboards. Buy child-proofing devices to attach to drawers and cabinet doors to make it hard for a child to open them.

Look up the telephone number of the nearest poison control center and post it next to the phone. Should an emergency occur, this will spare you the time it would take to look it up. Toll-free numbers are usually listed in the front of the phone book.

If you think a child has swallowed something poisonous, and seems very ill, call 911 or go to an emergency room immediately.

If you know what the substance is, and he does not seem ill, quickly give him water to drink to dilute the poison. While he is drinking the water, call a poison control center. According to the type of poison, you will be advised either to induce vomiting or to neutralize or dilute the substance in the stomach. *Do not guess.* Some poisons can do even greater damage when vomited.

If for some reason you are unable to reach a telephone, general guidelines are as follows.

For medicines and poisonous plants, vomiting should usually be induced right away, since the longer the substance is in the stomach, the more it will be absorbed and the more seriously ill the child will be. If any is still in his mouth, rinse or clear it out, then (if possible) hold the child upside down, with his head lower than his waist, and stick two fingers down his throat to cause the gag reflex. This will most likely bring up the contents of the stomach.

If he doesn't throw up right away, have him drink large amounts of lukewarm water and try again, or use syrup of ipecac according to the directions on the label. Or stir two tablespoons of mustard or salt into a glass of warm water and have him drink it. If he still does not throw up, take him to an emergency room to have his stomach pumped. Bring any remnants of the poison substance with you to help the hospital staff decide upon an antidote.

Some poisons, such as strong acids and alkalis, should *not* be vomited. They may burn the esophagus and throat so severely on the way back up that the tissues can be permanently scarred. For strong acids such as battery acid, or acids found among photographic chemicals, give the child cool water mixed with a spoonful of baking soda; baking soda is alkaline and will help to neutralize the acid. After this, give olive oil or milk to protect the stomach lining. Do not force these liquids down too quickly, or in too great quantities; you do not want the child to vomit.

Strong alkalis such as drain cleaners or oven cleaners should be diluted by drinking water mixed with lemon juice or vinegar (acids, which help neutralize the alkali), followed by milk or olive oil to protect the digestive tract.

Oily substances, and petroleum products such as gasoline, when vomited, form droplets that may be drawn into the lungs, causing problems much more severe than those that come from ingesting them. If a child has swallowed one of these, give him milk, or milk of magnesia—or water if that is all that is available—to neutralize or at least dilute the poison.

A tablespoonful of activated charcoal drunk down in a cup of water can help neutralize some poisons. The "universal antidote"—milk of magnesia, burnt toast, and strong tea—is sometimes helpful.

HERB TEAS. To help soothe and detoxify, after appropriate treatment of poisoning: Comfrey root, slippery elm, dandelion root.

HOMEOPATHIC REMEDIES.
> *Arsenicum album*—severe vomiting or diarrhea, burning pains, restlessness combined with great exhaustion.
> *Aconitum napellus*—the child is extremely frightened and agitated.
> *Cantharis*—intense burning pain, pale skin.
> *Carbo vegetabilis*—digestive upset, bloating; child may collapse, feel desperate for air.
> *Nux vomica*—for aftereffects of poisoning; child may feel sick, chilly, irritable.
> *Veratrum album*—great weakness, cold sweat, severe vomiting and diarrhea.

DRUGS AND MODERN MEDICAL PROCEDURES

Many of us who arc now parents grew up in the age of "wonder drugs" and "modern medical miracles." The more conscientious our schools and parents were, the more vaccinations and medications we probably had. Sick or not, we may have had our tonsils out, and many of us were screened for rare diseases with "harmless" X rays. We atc the latest in processed food, took fluoride drops, received rewards of lollipops, and respected the authorities who said that vitamins, health foods, and herbs were quackery. Perhaps the medical breakthroughs of the era spared us, here and there, from some diseases—but now that time has passed and brought us a wider perspective, we must ponder other questions. Are the chronic, alarming illnesses that limit so many adults today related to suppressive treatments received in childhood? Have the more invasive or chemical forms of health care popular since the 1950s contributed to present derangements of people's systems, setting them up for chronic fatigue, depression, allergies, spinal and nervous problems, autoimmune disorders, cancer, degenerative diseases, and immune insufficiencies?

It is not a matter of placing blame. If artificial medicine has done our generation harm, it is no one's fault. Most scientists and doctors of the time were sincere in using such techniques, and parents trusted science and tried to do what was best for the children. Now that we know of established (and suggested) dangers of chemicals and invasive therapeutic or diagnostic measures, if we subject our children to these it will be our responsibility.

There is not room in this book to discuss all medications and procedures prescribed by doctors and currently used in health care. Parents should be aware that most of these have side effects. If a drug is ever prescribed for your child, be sure to ask the reason for the prescription, what the drug's action is in the body, and what its dangers and side effects can be. The doctor should be able to give or show you detailed literature that explains these things. Although most doctors do their best, they are usually pressed for time and do not always learn or remember the actions of all available drugs or their side-effects. There are thousands of drugs produced in huge volume by pharmaceutical companies, and their salesmen avidly press doctors to buy and use them. This pressure may not be the doctor's fault, but it isn't yours (or your child's) either! Do not let your questions be pushed aside: the question of putting chemicals into your child's body is far from trivial. After asking the doctor, do your own independent reading as well. The *Physician's Desk Reference* (*PDR*) and other books on medical drugs can be found in the library reference section or bookstores. Decide on the basis of real information whether or not to accept and use a drug that has been prescribed. The following are often prescribed for children's illnesses.

ASPIRIN. Recommended for pain, inflammation, and fever reduction, aspirin is often thought of as benign and harmless. This is actually not the case. Among aspirin's possible side-effects are nausea, ringing in the ears, indigestion, rash, internal bleeding, and hives. The use of aspirin, especially for fever and viral illnesses, has been linked to a severe, encephalitis-like illness that can be deadly.

ACETAMINOPHEN. Often recommended for the same conditions as aspirin, acetaminophen (commonly known as Tylenol) is safer in that it has not been linked to Reye's syndrome. However, it still has side effects, and overdoses can cause serious liver damage, and large overdoses have been known to cause fatalities in very small children.

ANTIBIOTICS. Antibiotics, designed to enter the bloodstream and poison bacteria, are frequently prescribed by doctors for infections. Some physicians prescribe them "preventively" in viral conditions, in case a bacterial complication might later arise. Antibiotics are toxic and can be harmful to the body; they tax the liver and often disrupt digestion, causing nausea, diarrhea, and malabsorption of nutrients. Antibiotics are usually effective emergency medicines in very serious cases of infection such as bacterial pneumonia or meningitis; however, ideally their use should be restricted to such emergencies.

If you choose to have your child take antibiotics, watch carefully for any signs of allergic reaction: rashes, vomiting, headache, trouble breathing. Extra vitamin C, E, and B-complex should be given along with antibiotics to help reduce the toxic effects of the drug. (Some doctors, on request, will give a child intravenous vitamins C, B_6, and minerals along with antibiotics while fighting serious infection in the hospital.) Acidophilus culture, found in capsules, tablets, powders, liquids, and in cultured milk products such as yogurt or kefir, should be given every day during the course of medication and for two or three weeks afterward. This will help to preserve the growth of healthy bacteria in the intestines, since drugs that kill the bad bacteria also kill the good ones.

ANTIHISTAMINES. These drugs are used to block the inflammatory reaction set up by the body in response to infective agents, irritants, or allergens. They are often prescribed for simple symptoms such as nasal congestion, rashes, and swelling, or to help control nausea, motion sickness, tremor, or dizziness. Besides the fact that taking antihistamines in drug form may decrease the body's likelihood of creating natural antihistamine substances, many children experience side effects, such as nausea, vomiting, constipation, diarrhea, weakness, drowsiness, or overexcitability. Side effects of even small amounts are sometimes identical to symptoms of overdose; among these are dry mouth, palpitations, breathing problems, urinary retention, visual disturbances, and hallucinations. Many natural remedies are just as effective as antihistamines and do not have these dangers. (See sections on specific conditions in Part Three.)

STEROIDS. Corticosteroid drugs are usually prescribed for their anti-inflammatory or antiallergic actions. They are taken internally, or used in ointments on the skin. These drugs can upset the endocrine balance in the body, depress immune function, and interfere with growth and development. They can also interfere with carbohydrate, protein, and fat metabolism, the balance of water and minerals in the body, proper function of muscles and connective tissues, and contribute to blood or brain disorders. Because the use of steroids creates a drug dependency, a child who needs to stop taking them will have to have them withdrawn from his system gradually. Because of the dangers, parents should explore all avenues of alternative therapy instead of using steroids.

SURGERY. Surgery for children is, in certain cases, vital to survival or needed to correct very limiting problems or defects. It is important for parents to understand that any surgery, however simple the procedure, may be a risk to a child's life. Some children undergoing operations for minor problems have died from improper anesthesia or have contracted serious infections in the hospital. Unless the need is obvious, get several opinions if a doctor recommends surgery for your child. (For the best perspective on the problem, try to choose doctors who work in different medical centers and are not acquainted with each other.) If your child truly needs an operation, find a doctor who has performed the specific procedure successfully many times. Try to find parents of children who have had the same type of operation and can recommend a doctor. Try also to find a hospital in which children's surgery is performed frequently, with anesthesiologists well-practiced in correct administration of anesthetics for children.

If the need for surgery is not completely clear, explore more natural alternatives. Homeopathic physicians, chiropractors, naturopaths, and acupuncturists are sometimes able to correct conditions for which the only allopathic treatment is surgery.

X RAYS. The dangers of X rays are now more widely known than they were several decades ago, but this does not mean that doctors are cautious enough in prescribing them. Seeing an image of the body's internal structures can be helpful to a doctor making a diagnosis, but radiation is cumulative and ultimately dangerous. X ray should not be used, especially on growing children, unless it is absolutely justified. If a fracture of a bone or a serious internal defect is suspected, X rays may be justified. X rays are not justified when used to check for minor problems, or conditions such as pneumonia or constipation in which the information gained from the X ray picture would not change the course of treatment significantly. If the doctor wants to take X rays, ask him or her to explain exactly why they are necessary. Tell the doctor you don't want your child exposed to needless radiation. Remind the doctor that diagnostic X rays taken in the past at levels then considered safe are now considered the cause of certain cases of cancer; levels *now* considered safe may some day be considered dangerous. If a child really needs an X ray taken, make sure all other parts of the body are protected by a lead apron and special shields. Give extra vitamins C and E and kelp (for several days before the X ray if possible, and for the following week) to help protect the child's body tissues against the radiation.

IMMUNIZATIONS

The subject of immunization is a very important one and increasingly controversial. The concept of giving simple, safe, almost painless injections—and thereby protecting children from serious, potentially crippling or fatal diseases—is extremely appealing. The world is an uncertain place, and, especially in regard to the health of our own beloved children, parents are ready to rush for whatever can promise safety. However, as is the case with so many other important issues in life, immunization is not as safe or simple as its theorists had hoped. Vaccines vary widely in effectiveness and purity, even from batch to batch; they do not always adequately protect against the diseases for which they have been developed, and some have very serious side effects.

The theory behind immunizations is, in simple terms, that when vaccines containing diluted or altered forms of bacteria, viruses, or their toxic products are introduced into a child's body, the immune system is given a chance to develop recognition of—and therefore resistance to—the disease agent, without becoming infected by the disease itself. The development of this recognition, and the production of antibodies specific to the substances in the vaccine, are thought to enable the body to easily resist the real disease in case the child is later exposed to it.

The benefits and dangers of immunization seem partly to be determined by the constitution, immune function, and sensitivity of the individual child. All children are different; it is hard to know in advance how a four-month-old infant will respond to the injection of a foreign substance. There is no risk-free answer to the immunization question, but when parents are faced with deciding whether or not to have their child immunized, they may want to consider the following information.

Diphtheria, pertussis (whooping cough), tetanus, and polio are the diseases for which immunizations are most firmly recommended by doctors and public health agencies. (Vaccines for the first three are often administered together as "DPT.") All of these diseases can be serious, life-threatening conditions. They are also fairly rare. Some experts think that immunizations are responsible for the decline in these diseases; some do not. It is true that diphtheria, pertussis, tetanus, and polio are not as common today as they were before the institution of immunization programs, but there is evidence that improved nutrition, housing conditions, and sanitation have played a large part in their decline.

Some diseases are thought by scientists to cyclically increase and decrease in virulence, for reasons unrelated to immunization. For instance, scarlet fever, which was once considered an extremely dangerous disease, and for which there is no vaccine, is now much less dangerous than it was a hundred years ago. There is evidence that the incidence of diphtheria was on the decline before any vaccine for it was developed. There is also indication that large numbers of children all over the world—immunized and unimmunized—become infected with the polio virus, get flulike symptoms, and get over them in a few days without the disease ever becoming severe enough to warrant a doctor's visit

The vaccines, although designed to prevent particular diseases, do not always confer immunity. There are many people who have been "fully immunized" who have shown little or no immunity to these diseases when tested. People immunized against specific diseases nevertheless often catch them during epidemics. In part, this may be due to some batches of vaccine distributed to doctors and clinics not being as well manufactured or as effective as others. There are also other factors in the health of individuals equally important to, or more important than, immunization. Many people who are not vaccinated against these diseases are exposed to them and do *not* catch them. People whose resistance is low because of other illnesses, inadequate shelter, or poor nutrition are more likely to become seriously ill when exposed.

Common side effects are swelling at the injection sight, irritibility, and low-grade fever. More serious side effects, which should be reported to a doctor, are prolonged screaming, limpness or paleness, fever higher than 102°, shock, and encephalitis. All of these side effects have occurred within minutes, hours, days, or weeks of receiving the shot. A substantial number of sudden unexplained infant deaths (SIDS, or "crib-deaths") occur within a week of DPT and polio immunizations. Although the shots are not considered to be the actual cause of SIDS, there are physicians who believe that the resulting stress on the immune system may be a factor in those infants who already had a pre-disposition to SIDS.

The pertussis portion of the DPT vaccine is the one most likely to cause dramatic adverse reactions. It is also the least effective component of the vaccine. In many parts of Europe, the pertussis portion has been removed from immunization programs after careful weighing of the risks and benefits.

MMR (measles, mumps, rubella) immunization for children is also highly recommended by many clinics and doctors. These diseases are sometimes serious but rarely life-threatening, and few cases are severe or dangerously complicated in children who were well cared-for while ill and not debilitated before coming down with the illness. There are some exceptions: measles can cause deafness due to encephalitis or nerve damage. Similar problems also occur as reactions to measles vaccine.

Rubella is a mild disease in children, but is considered dangerous because of the devastating birth defects it can cause when contracted by pregnant women. Because of this, many doctors feel that rubella ought to be eradicated through vaccination. The question is, *does* the vaccine eradicate it? Sadly, there is evidence that the immunity to rubella supposedly conferred by vaccination can diminish as the years go by, and that women who had rubella shots as children and think themselves immune can catch it later at an age at which they're far more likely to be pregnant. Since having the actual disease of rubella appears to give lifelong immunity, some experts feel that rubella-related birth defects would be better prevented by making sure that little girls are exposed to rubella until they catch it, rather than having the shots.

A chicken pox vaccine has recently been developed made of the live weakened virus *Varicella zoster,* thought to cause both chicken pox and shingles. It is unclear at this time how long the immunity will last, whether it will wear off and those immunized as children may later catch chicken pox at an age when it can be more serious, or whether the "silent" virus in the body will lead to the painful condition of shingles in later life. Any new vaccine or medication should be investigated closely. Vaccines and medications are tested on limited groups of subjects, and are often too quickly judged safe by their researchers and manufacturers and then endorsed by well-meaning physicians who believe the literature; it is only later, after widespread use, that the dangers and long-term effects of vaccines may become apparent.

Other possible effects of immunization are being investigated by health researchers. Among these are: an overall decline in a child's health after receiving shots; the onset of illnesses similar to the diseases the shots were designed to prevent, but with some of the symptoms masked or changed; derangements of the immune system; autoimmune diseases such as multiple sclerosis and lupus, many of which were not recognized until after immunizations were introduced; damage to the central nervous system, and changes in brain tissue suspected of being connected with hyperactivity, learning problems, and criminal behavior. The connections between these problems and immunizations have not been firmly established, but they should continue to be investigated. Those of us who care about the health and happiness of children hope that the truth is discovered, whatever it is. The point in exploring the risks of vaccines is certainly not to untruthfully blame problems on them; however, since the issue involved in immunization is the protection of children's health and life, no possible links or risks should be ignored.

Other risks from vaccines may be due to industrial practices. Vaccines are sometimes produced and marketed whose ingredients are in inappropriate or unsafe proportions. Toxic substances such as formaldehyde (a carcinogen), mercury (a toxic metal), phenol, acetone, and aluminum phosphate are sometimes found in vaccines. No one knows for certain what effects these chemicals might have when injected into babies or small children, whose brains and bodies are developing rapidly. Sometimes batches of vaccine become contaminated, some have been made from inferior or ineffective materials, some have been improperly formulated—yet mistakes such as these have been missed at the laboratory, and faulty vaccines released to doctors and clinics.

Parents are frequently not given thorough information about the side effects and risks of vaccines. Many parents are still unaware that DPT, MMR, and other shots have real dangers. I have conversed with many workers at well-baby clinics, public health nurses, and pediatricians who express the belief that to raise the issue of bad vaccine reactions is needlessly upsetting. Parents who bring their children in for shots are usually given leaflets that tell of potential side effects, are asked to sign a paper stating their informed consent and, if they express alarm, are often told that they "worry too much," that a bad reaction only happens to "one in a thousand"—as if this assured them that their precious child will not be that "one."

It is not always emphasized strongly enough to parents that certain aspects of their family medical history, such as seizure disorders, aneurysms, allergies, parents or siblings with shot reactions, may put their healthy children at serious risk if they are immunized. Too many have found this out the hard way. Among my patients and friends are families whose lives have been changed irrevocably because they "responsibly" took their children in for shots and, as a result, those children are now debilitated, paralyzed, blind, epileptic, retarded, or brain damaged.

Immunization of children is required by law in most of the United States, and children are required to be up to date with their shots to attend public schools. Those who have religious objections are sometimes exempted from pressure to have their children immunized. Children who have had extreme reactions to previous shots are sometimes, but not always, excused. Because of the laws and pressures, parents are made to feel that they really don't have much choice. They *want* to trust their doctors and the government, and so are persuaded to think that immunizations must be all right.

Some doctor's choose to downplay immunization's dangers to ensure that parents follow the vaccination program. Although most of these doctor's honestly believe in the benefits of immunizations, they should still give parents all the information, including the risk factors involved, and then respect the parent's right to decide. Parents should be aware that whether or not they choose to have their chidren immunized they are taking a risk, but they need to be as informed as possible in order to make a responsible decision. Even if the odds of severe reactions are low, children are not statistics to their parents. And yet, conscientious parents are too often made to feel that their doubts and questions are extreme and foolish.

Many health practitioners both of allopathic and naturopathic bent, label as "biased" persons who bring the risks and potential risks of immunizations to light. Physicians with such views should remember that the primary precept for doctors is "to do no harm." This means that the safety of drugs and procedures, including vaccines, cannot be decided by percentages and odds, or by finance and politics. If immunization is dangerous, even to only a handful of children, those children have a right to be protected from illness and damage, and a safer alternative must be sought.

POSSIBLE ALTERNATIVES. Parents and physicians must press the government to fund the development of truly safe vaccines, or to support research into other methods of protection. They should write to their representatives in Congress and tell them that they will adamantly refuse to have their children immunized until there is a safe alternative.

Vaccine manufacturers must be compelled to screen vaccines more carefully so that none are contaminated or improperly prepared. Parents and physicians should write letters to members of Congress, demanding that the government put such pressure on the manufacturers.

Families of some of the children who have been damaged or killed by vaccine are being awarded monetary compensation. Those who qualify must have had the reactions between certain dates and must file within a certain amount of time. These limits have been set, apparently, to financially protect the government and vaccine manufacturers. Parents who disagree with these limitations should write to members of Congress and express their views.

PRACTICAL MEASURES. If you decide to have your child immunized, there are some precautions you can take to help prevent a bad reaction.

Giving extra vitamin C, A, E, and B-complex, calcium, and magnesium every day for a week before the shots may help the child's system deal with the stress and the injected foreign substance.

Echinacea tea, several cups a day, before and after the shot may help.

Homeopathic treatment of reaction to immunizations is often effective. The remedy must be prescribed individually, according to the symptoms that the child shows. (See the chapter on Homeopathy in Part One and FEVER in Part Three.) In case of a serious reaction, seek emergency medical care as well as the help of an experienced homeopath.

Some homeopathic physicians give remedies called *nosodes* as an alternative to vaccination for serious diseases. These are made of much more dilute and potentized substances than regular vaccines and do not have dangerous side effects. Documented cases indicate that giving nosodes to exposed people has decreased the rate of contraction or severity of certain diseases in times of epidemic, but whether they actually give children long-term protection against the diseases if taken in lieu of immunization is not yet clear. Research into the possible benefits of nosodes should be funded and pursued. Parents should use political and personal pressure to insist that such nontoxic and possibly efficacious avenues be honestly and thoroughly explored.

Information about the pros and cons of immunization can be found in several books and booklets, among which are the following: Randall Neustaedter's *The Immunization Decision* (Berkeley: North Atlantic Books, 1991); Dr. Robert Mendelsohn's *How to Raise a Healthy Child . . . In Spite of Your Doctor* (New York: Ballantine, 1987); Barbara Loe Fisher and Dr. Harris L. Coulter's *DPT: A Shot in the Dark* (New York: Warner Books, 1986), and Dr. Robert Moskowitz's pamphlet, *The Case Against Immunizations*, available from The National Center for Homeopathy, 1500 Massachusettes Avenue, NW, Washington, D.C., 20005. See also Dr. Robert Mendelsohn's newsletters on immunization (available from "The People's Doctor," 664 North Michigan Avenue, Suite 720, Chicago, Illinois, 60611); and the *Mothering* magazine article, "Immunizations: Mothering Special Edition," available by writing Mothering Magazine, in New Mexico.

PART 3
A I L M E N T S

Abdominal Pain

Abdominal pain in children usually comes from some disorder in the workings of the stomach or intestines. Common causes are emotional tension, indigestion, overeating, gas, constipation, food allergy, food poisoning, ingestion of a nonfood substance, poisoning, and reaction to medication. If the reason for discomfort is not obvious and the child seems very unwell, consider the following possible conditions (and refer to the corresponding section in this book).

APPENDICITIS
Pain and tenderness may start near the navel, and later move to the lower right part of the abdomen. This pain is not made better by passing gas or having a bowel movement. There is often some fever but it is not necessarily high, and there may be nausea and loss of appetite. The child may lie with his right leg bent; flexing it against his abdomen may be very painful. He may also find it hard to stand on his right leg and support the weight of his body. The possibility of appendicitis should be considered, especially if other members of the family have had it, since there seems to be some familial predisposition.

INTESTINAL OBSTRUCTION
Pain in the abdomen is very severe and cramplike. It occurs at intervals, which become shorter and shorter as time goes by. Sometimes there is violent vomiting. There might be odd bowel movements with blood in them, bloody mucus discharged, or no bowel movements at all. A fast pulse, cold hands and feet and cold sweat, dehydration, and collapse may eventually occur. This is an extreme emergency. Any child with these symptoms should have medical care at once.

HEPATITIS
Pain is felt in the upper right side of the abdomen, with flulike symptoms: nausea, vomiting, fever, dark urine and, after several days, jaundice (seen as yellowing of the skin and eyewhites).

URINARY TRACT INFECTION
Symptoms may seem like severe flu; pain may be felt in the lower back, radiating into the lower abdomen and groin. The urine is

scanty, cloudy or dark, and sometimes painful to pass. Face and ankles can be swollen and puffy. Analysis of urine for bacteria, pus, or blood can determine whether infection exists.

Other conditions that may cause abdominal pain include allergy, celiac disease (see WEIGHT PROBLEMS), colds, colic, constipation, dehydration, diabetes, diarrhea, emotional tension, flu, food poisoning, gas, hernia, injury to internal organs such as the liver or spleen from a blow or a fall, swollen lymph nodes because of illness or infection, side effects of medication, menstrual cramps, muscle strain of the abdominal or pelvic muscles, nutritional deficiencies or indiscretions, poisoning, stomach disorders such as ulcers, and worms.

Any unexplained, persistent abdominal discomfort should have the attention of a physician to make sure the cause is nothing serious.

WHAT A PHYSICIAN MAY DO

A physician will examine the child's abdomen, and probably also her chest, ears, and throat. The doctor may do a rectal exam. Blood and urine samples may be taken and analyzed. If a particular condition (such as intestinal obstruction) is suspected, the doctor may want to perform special diagnostic procedures, such as giving a barium enema and taking X rays.

WHAT YOU CAN DO AT HOME

PRACTICAL MEASURES. With any sort of abdominal pain, help the child be as comfortable and relaxed as possible. Some may want to lie quietly in bed; some want to be held; some need to sit up and do something.

To find out whether the condition is serious, gently touch the child's abdomen, checking for tender or rigid places. Ask questions (without too pointedly suggesting answers) to find out as clearly as possible what the pain is like and how severe it is, as well as any other symptoms. The information you collect in this way will be useful to the doctor or health care professional, if you decide to call one; a doctor may be able to advise you over the phone and spare you the strain and expense of a trip to the office or emergency room.

For information on nutrition, herbs, homeopathic remedies, and acupressure points for abdominal pain, see APPENDICITIS, CONSTIPATION, DIARRHEA, INDIGESTION AND GAS, and NAUSEA AND VOMITING.

ACNE

Teenagers and children near the age of puberty usually, to their chagrin, find blackheads and pimples popping out on face, neck, chest, back and other areas. These are places that are well supplied with sebaceous glands, which provide lubricating oil for the skin. As sex hormones begin to be produced, these glands are stimulated to overproduce oil, and the pores of the skin become clogged and sometimes infected. Moderate acne does not mean that the child is particularly unhealthy; very few teenagers escape without the occasional crop of pimples. But many teenagers feel that any flaw in physical appearance is an emergency. Because of this, parents should be prepared to provide emotional support, and information about natural measures that will help keep their children away from drastic and dangerous skin treatments.

The bacteria involved in acne are normal bacteria: that is, bacteria that are always present on healthy skin. It is not the existence of these microorganisms that causes the infection, but the skin's impaired resistance to them. This underlying weakness in the skin's resistance may be due to emotional stresses, nutritional inadequacies, overindulgence in nonnutritious foods, allergies, reactions to medications, or improper skin care.

Blackheads are not black because of dirt but because of a chemical change that takes place in the oil in the pores when exposed to air. Moderate washing, especially when the skin is actually dirty, is helpful, but scrubbing and disinfecting can be overdone and will remove the natural protective oil from the skin, making it more susceptible to infection. Squeezing blackheads and pimples is hard to resist, but, especially on the face, this pastime may bruise the tissue and make it more likely to become infected. Using a pin or other unsterilized instrument can lead to serious infection and scarring.

WHAT A PHYSICIAN MAY DO

Doctors may recommend medications called exfoliates—which keep the follicles open and encourage skin cells and oil to ooze out—or over-the-counter drying agents. Antibiotics such as tetracycline or chloramphenicol are often prescribed to kill the bacteria that live in pimples, especially in cases of deep acne where cysts have formed. This course of treatment can reduce the amount of active infection, but it is only removing the symptoms, not correcting the cause. Such drugs may be recommended for daily use over months or even years. There is a need for caution, as antibiotics may have side effects such as stomach pain, colitis, or depression of the bone marrow, which lowers the child's immune function. It has also become apparent that frequent use of antibiotics may lead to dangerous drug allergy or systemic yeast infection (candidiasis).

Another drug used for acne is isotretinoin, or Accutane (a toxic derivative of vitamin A), whose side effects include inflammation of mucous membranes, hair loss, and elevated triglyceride and cholesterol levels. Hormones, corticosteroids, abrasion of the skin, and even X rays have been used on occasion to combat teenage acne. Such treatments may temporarily affect the symptoms but often do no lasting good, and some have been known to contribute to enzyme disorders, hormonal imbalances, liver damage, or cancer.

Some teenagers are so conscious of their appearance that they may be inclined to risk anything to get rid of skin troubles. The emotional force may be so great that the child cannot be reasonable in choosing a treatment. If so, understanding parents will try to provide safe alternatives to dangerous or suppressive medical procedures, and to help the child control his diet and habits, rather than knowingly let him risk his health.

If the acne is dangerously infected and extremely painful, look for a physician who treats skin problems by purifying the system and strengthening it against infection, rather than one who uses drugs or drastic therapies.

WHAT YOU CAN DO AT HOME

NUTRITION. The child's diet should be kept free of refined and processed foods, concentrated sweets, fried or highly spicy dishes, beef, and alcohol. Lots of vegetables and fruits should be provided, especially cucumbers, green peppers, carrots, celery, beets, and apricots. Fish, brown rice, oatmeal, soy products, and sunflower and sesame seeds are also beneficial. Eliminating wheat or dairy products is often effective. Iodized salt should be avoided. The possibility of food allergy should be considered: even healthful foods can contribute to skin problems if the child is allergic to them. (See ALLERGIES.) The child should drink several quarts of liquid daily—fruit or vegetable juices, water, mild herb teas (and *no* sodas full of sugar or caffeine) to help her system rid itself of impurities.

Vitamins A, E, C, B-complex (including choline, inositol, biotin, niacin and pantothenic acid), beta carotene, calcium, magnesium, and zinc are especially needed during outbreaks of acne. Omega-3 and omega-6 fatty acids have been known to help. (See the chapter on Nutrition in Part One.)

HERB TEAS. Red clover, echinacea, calendula.

NATURAL APPLICATIONS. Poultices of grated cucumber or carrot may be applied to the skin for half an hour a day to draw out impurities. Cosmetic clay (bentonite) may be used the same way. Skin-washes made of peppermint, yarrow root, lavender, or comfrey (brewed as tea and cooled) are helpful. Dabbing aloe vera, lemon, cucumber juice, or vitamin E on the spots a few times a day can help clear them up.

Sunlight in moderation, fresh air, and a cheerful and relaxing atmosphere are generally beneficial. Self-consciousness, brooding, rebellion, and lack of confidence are often part of the transition to adulthood; parents should try to keep in touch with teenage family members in a friendly, open way, to reduce the pressures on their children and on themselves.

HOMEOPATHIC REMEDIES. In cases of serious acne, a constitutional remedy that fits the individual child is recommended. (See the Homeopathy chapter in Part One.) Help should be sought from an experienced homeopathic prescriber. If this is not possible, one of the following remedies may help.

Antimonium tartaricum. Long-lasting acne with many large pustules.
Calcarea carbonica. Acne in a child who is overweight, clammy, craves sweets.

Hepar sulphuris calcareum. Painful boils slow to come to a head; child is chilly and irritable.

Kali bromatum. Itching acne; child has restless sleep, nightmares, depression.

Silicea. Deep acne; hard, swollen glands; child has headaches, is tired, nervous.

Sulphur. Red, rough, burning eruptions, aggravated by washing; child may crave sweets and spicy food.

ACUPRESSURE AND MASSAGE. (See Acupressure Appendix for directions.)

LU 1: A tender point in the indentation below the shoulder end of the collarbone.

LV 14: A tender point on the front of the rib cage, midway between the nipple and the lower ribs.

LI 4: The point at the end of the crease between the thumb and index finger.

LV 3: A tender point midway between the first and second metatarsal bones.

ALLERGIES

An allergy is a sensitivity to a particular substance, causing an overreaction of the immune system. The offending agent may be inhaled, ingested, injected, or come into contact with skin or mucous membranes. When exposed to allergens, the body responds by releasing varying amounts of histamine and other mediators of inflammation from body tissues. The symptoms produced by allergy include rashes, swelling, hives, runny nose, congestion, asthma, vomiting, dark circles under the eyes, pallor, diarrhea, intestinal bleeding, muscle spasms, and—in severe cases— suffocation, unconsciousness, and shock. It is common for people to suffer from hidden chronic allergies of which they are unaware. Although reactions are not instantaneous and dramatic, these allergies may decrease the person's energy, cause mood swings, and reduce resistance to disease.

Hay fever is an allergy to pollens and therefore, unless compounded by other allergies, occurs in particular seasons. Other common allergens are dust, animal hair and dander, insects (such as fleas or dust mites), smoke, feathers, molds, wool, synthetic materials, bedding (pillow or mattress stuffing), plants (poison oak, poison ivy), dyes, metals such as nickel (found in jewelry, braces, dental fillings), cosmetics, soaps, shampoos, medications, pesticides, preservatives, pollutants, food additives, and certain foods. Some persons respond allergically to extremes in temperature. Acute allergic reactions may resemble head colds, with a rundown feeling, sneezing, irritated eyes, runny nose, and clear, watery discharge. Green or yellow discharge often indicates a bacterial infection such as sinusitis, tonsillitis, or bronchitis, to which allergy can make the person more susceptible.

A tendency to allergies often runs in families, but may be caused or increased by emotional stress, low blood sugar, inadequate liver function (often because of overexposure to pollutants or chemicals), nutritional deficiencies, overworked adrenal glands, or low production of digestive enzymes.

FOOD ALLERGY

Feeding cow's milk or formula to an infant rather than breast feeding is thought to contribute to a child's tendency toward food allergy. So is introduction of solid food into a baby's diet too soon. Small babies do not have the enzymes and digestive juices needed to completely break down food for proper absorption. Incompletely broken-down food elements are read by the child's body as foreign substances, triggering an inflammatory response. The child's immune system then recognizes the substance as an invader and responds allergically each time it is encountered.

Symptoms of food allergy may show up within minutes of eating the offending food, or at any time up to a week later. Symptoms include: stomachache, nausea, diarrhea, runny nose, coughing, wheezing, hives, rashes, or eczema; in extreme cases, anaphylactic shock may occur (see Emergencies chapter in Part Two). Food allergies beginning in infancy are frequently overcome as a child gets older, but many remain on some level for the rest of the person's life.

Foods to which people are often allergic are milk and dairy products, gluten-containing grains such as wheat, rye, barley (or breads made from other grains with gluten added), eggs, citrus fruits, beef, veal, fish, nuts, shellfish, tomatoes, pork, strawberries, chocolate, and certain cheeses. Refined sugar and processed foods may exaggerate a child's tendency to react allergically. Children are often sensitive to additives like artificial sweeteners, sulfites, dyes, and monosodium glutamate (MSG).

It has been noted that a person often craves foods that contain some nutrient his system desperately needs; for instance, people who crave chocolate often really need its magnesium. Unfortunately, a person may also crave foods to which he is allergic. Such cravings may, however, be a clue to use in tracking down the allergen.

WHAT A PHYSICIAN MAY DO

Health care professionals vary vastly in their attitude toward, diagnosis of, and treatment for allergies. Some try to detect allergens by use of blood tests (such as RAST or cytotoxic testing), patch or scratch tests on the skin, double-blind challenge, muscle tests, or pulse tests. Some tend to find many allergies of varying severity in the patient and prescribe a rigorous and complicated regimen; others find only one or two allergens and simply recommend avoiding them.

Doctors often prescribe antihistamines to remove allergy symptoms, sometimes recommending that the drugs be taken before an attack occurs. Because antihistamines are not curing the physical weakness that causes the allergy—only taking away certain symptoms—this sort of treatment is of limited use and dangerous because such drugs may have toxic side effects and may make the child's system even less likely to overcome the allergy by itself.

Some physicians treat allergic individuals through *hyposensitization,* a procedure that consists of injecting very small amounts of the trigger substance underneath the skin. The amounts are gradually increased until the person's system gets used to the exposure and reactions to the substance become mild. For some patients this works very well, some are helped in part, and others not at all. The idea of receiving an injection once a week for months or even years is not likely to be appealing to a child, so the pros and cons should be weighed carefully.

For food allergy, restrictive eliminative diets and rotation diets are usually recommended. If you need an expert's guidance, try to find a physician whose approach and temperament suit your child's personality and special needs. A course of treatment works only if the patient *follows* it.

WHAT YOU CAN DO AT HOME

If your child shows many allergy-related problems, has low energy, and is often ill, her general health and resistance need to be improved. No matter how many tests are done to determine which specific substances are allergens, it is only by strengthening the child's system that the allergy will be overcome. A tendency toward allergy may be hereditary; however, pregnant or nursing women who maintain well-balanced diets of natural, chemical-free foods, vary their protein sources, and consume only small amounts of foods that tend to induce allergy, will decrease the chances that their children will be allergic.

PRACTICAL MEASURES. Keep the child from being exposed to any substance that seems to bring on allergic symptoms, fatigue, or mood changes. If you don't know what triggers the reaction, try to eliminate strong suspects from the environment or diet. If the allergy symptoms seem to clear up within several days, reintroduce the suspects one by one (a new one every few days); should a reaction appear, the latest substance is likely to be an offender. Do this in a systematic way, as it is quite possible that the person is allergic to more than one thing.

The emotional factors in this type of regimen must be considered. If the child seems to be allergic to the family pet, try to arrange a compromise: animals should not be allowed in the child's room, and should be groomed and played with outdoors if possible. If a child appears to have multiple food allergies, do not be too restrictive in your search for the offenders; try to find special, tasty foods that she can have (such as nondairy ice creams, wheat-free cookies, or rice snacks) and try to reward her for her patience with extra attention, toys, or outings.

Try to keep stress factors in the child's environment to a minimum. Do not smoke or use strong toxic or fumy substances in the house. Vacuum regularly to minimize dust and keep the house dry, well aired and free of molds. Use air filters and dehumidifiers if necessary. Try to make sure the emotional atmosphere is clear as well: give your child a chance to express her feelings and try not to overload her with responsibilities or criticism.

NUTRITION. Improve the child's diet in order to strengthen the liver, mucous membranes lining the digestive and respiratory tracts, and immune system. Because they are growing, children always need high-quality proteins, fresh fruits and vegetables, and adequate amounts of vitamins and minerals. When they show signs of allergy, their general nutritional needs are increased. Do not give your child any refined foods or foods with chemical additives. Try to provide good, clean, chemical-free protein sources such as fish, chicken, tofu, eggs, beans, and dairy products, making sure to use only those to which the child shows no sign of a bad reaction. Make sure nuts, seeds, and untreated vegetable oils are included to provide necessary unsaturated fatty acids. It is essential to detect and eliminate possible allergens, but it is also important, and sometimes brain-racking, to find alternatives that your child *will eat.* Cultured dairy products and certified raw milk seem to be tolerated by many children who react to regular grocery store milk; acidophilus (the benign bacteria in yogurt and kefir) is said to prevent putrefaction of food substances in the intestines and thereby reduce the production of histamine. Natural food stores and an increasing number of regular grocery stores sell wheat-free breads and snacks that contain no sugar or preservatives; some carry soy-based cheeses and ice cream made of soy or brown rice.

Don't be too strict about mealtimes. It is often better for a child to have many small meals a day than to have three large ones; this helps the blood-sugar level stay steady which helps stave off allergic reactions.

Vitamins A, C, E, and B-complex including pantothenic acid, manganese, magnesium, zinc, bioflavonoids, and beta carotene are especially helpful to the system of a child with allergies. (See Nutrition in Part One.)

Papaya enzyme tablets taken with meals can benefit protein digestion. Bee pollen granules can be taken with meals to help build resistance to some allergies. Start with one granule, and increase the number by one each day until reaching a teaspoonful per day. (If the pollen itself seems to bring on an allergic reaction, discontinue it.)

HERB TEAS. Red clover, mullein, goldenrod, coltsfoot, licorice root. (See also ASTHMA.)

HOMEOPATHIC REMEDIES. Deep-acting constitutional remedies are most useful to strengthen the defenses of allergic individuals. The following remedies can help reduce symptoms in acute situations.

Ferrum phosphoricum. May prevent or reduce the severity of an allergy attack, if taken as soon as symptoms begin.

Allium cepa. Red, watery eyes, clear nasal discharge that burns the skin, tickling cough, and sneezing; child is worse indoors, in warm rooms, and may be thirsty.

Arsenicum album. Discharge from the nose is watery and burns; child feels a tickling in the nose and may feel exhausted.

Euphrasia. Watery, irritated eyes, bland nose discharge, and coughed-up mucus; child may feel worse outdoors and in the morning, and more stuffy lying down.

Gelsemium. Child feels heavy and tired, has a headache at the back of the skull, and chills along the spine.

Natrum muriaticum. Nasal discharge is clear, like egg white; loss of taste or smell; child may be weepy or withdrawn and dislike consolation.

Nux vomica. Nose is alternately stuffed up (especially outdoors and at night) and runny (especially indoors and by day), with a teasing cough; throat feels scraped, tickly; child is irritable, chilly.

Sabadilla. Itching in nose, watery eyes and nose, sneezing spasms, sensation of a lump in the throat; child feels better outdoors in open air.

Wyethia. Intolerable itching of the roof of the mouth and behind the nose; child's nose is runny, but everything feels dry.

Apis mellifica. In cases of allergic shock, the symptoms of which include extreme swelling and difficulty breathing, this remedy has been known to save lives.

Carbolicum acidum. For allergic shock, if *Apis* does not work. The face may be dark or red, with pallor around the mouth.

ACUPRESSURE AND MASSAGE. *For all types of allergic conditions:*

LV14: A tender point on the front of the rib cage, midway between the nipple and the lower ribs.

LV 3: A tender point midway between the first and second metatarsal bones.

SP 6: A tender point three of the child's finger breadths above the inner anklebone.

ST 36: A tender point next to the outer side of the big bump at the top of the shin.

LI 4: The point at the end of the crease between the thumb and index finger.

Especially for allergies with head and respiratory symptoms:

LI 20: The tender points where the creases of the cheek meet the nose.

GB 20: A tender point in the muscles just below the base of the skull, midway between the central bump on the lower back of the head and the ear tip.

LI 11: A point at the end of the elbow-crease (thumb side) when the arm is bent.

LU 1: A tender point in the indentation below the shoulder end of the collarbone.

GB 14: A point on either side of the forehead, midway between eyebrow and hairline.

ANEMIA

Anemia is a condition in which the number of red blood cells, or the amount of hemoglobin present in red blood cells, is not sufficient. Hemoglobin, an iron-containing protein molecule, is responsible for carrying oxygen to all body tissues. If cells do not receive sufficient oxygen, their functioning is impaired, leading to tiredness, illness, or even death. The most common form of anemia in children is caused by iron deficiency. This is usually due to a dietary lack of iron, or to a problem with absorption of iron from the digestive tract; a child may fall behind nutritionally during periods of growth and become anemic. Deficiencies of copper, cobalt, or vitamin C, all of which play parts in iron assimilation, can also contribute to an anemic state. Sufficient folic acid and vitamin

B_{12} are needed for hemoglobin production; children on strict vegetarian diets may become anemic due to deficient B_{12} (pernicious anemia), or due to protein deficiency. Anemia can also be the result of blood loss from injury (internal or external) or bleeding in the digestive tract due to ulcers, tumors, allergic reactions, or excessive use of aspirin. Hereditary blood disorders (such as sickle cell disease and thalassemia), cancers, hypothyroidism, rheumatic fever, long-term infections, bone marrow dysfunction, radiation, and drug toxicity may also lead to anemia. Very heavy menstrual periods and anorexia and bulimia may also be associated with an anemic state.

An anemic child may exhibit one or many of the following symptoms: fatigue and disinclination to walk, difficulty using muscles, weakness, pale skin and lips, irritability, breathlessness (breath-holding in infants), dizziness, ringing in the ears, rapid heartbeats, night sweats, pica (a craving to eat dirt, clay starch, or ice), loss of appetite, nausea, and diarrhea. In addition to the above, a flabby, sore tongue, sore gums, weight loss, and tingling or numbness in the extremities may be signs of either folic acid deficiency or B_{12} deficiency.

WHAT A PHYSICIAN MAY DO
To be sure the symptoms are not caused by something more serious than simple iron deficiency, the doctor will check the child's heart, lungs, ears, nose, throat, and eyes for signs of infection, hookworm, or other problems. A blood sample may be taken to assess the percentage of blood made up of red blood cells (this ratio is known as the hematocrit) and the amount of hemoglobin carried by the blood.

Doctors usually treat anemia by advising improvement of the diet. Some will also prescribe an iron supplement. Be cautious about using these, especially ferrous sulfate; iron supplements can be toxic and may destroy vitamin E, which is needed for efficient use of oxygen. Ferrous gluconate is a safer compound, used in moderation, but iron is really more efficiently absorbed from foods. Some practitioners recommend supplements of other vitamins and minerals (B-complex with B_{12} and folic acid, vitamins C and E, cobalt and copper). Some may give betaine hydrochloride to improve digestion and food absorption and thus increase the amount of usable iron in the child's system.

Blood tests are used to distinguish between types of anemia unless the child's symptoms and dietary habits make the distinction clear. Vitamin B_{12} or folic acid supplements may be given if a deficiency is found. However, care must be taken with folic acid supplements; excess folic acid can mask B_{12} deficiency symptoms.

If the child's anemia is a result of blood loss or other disorders rather than dietary deficiency, the doctor will attempt to correct the cause. In extreme cases, blood transfusions may be given. In these days of AIDS and hepatitis, care must be taken that the blood used for transfusion is safe. The tests used to determine the purity of blood samples are not infallible, and there is always a possibility that blood may contain disease-causing elements for which there is as yet no test. If the child's blood type is compatible with that of a healthy family member, that person may be able to provide the needed blood.

WHAT YOU CAN DO AT HOME

PRACTICAL MEASURES. For prevention of anemia, nurse your infant if possible. Children who have been primarily bottle-fed or whose diets have consisted mostly of cow's milk are often found to be anemic between one and two years of age. Breast milk has more iron than cow's milk, in a form that is more easily absorbed.

Make sure the child does not drink coffee, black tea, or cola drinks that contain caffeine; caffeine and other substances in such drinks interfere with iron absorption. Cut down on milk products, as they can cause microscopic bleeding in the digestive tract. Avoid aspirin for the same reason.

NUTRITION. Whatever the origin of an anemic condition, while the cause must be corrected it is vital to strengthen the system through nutrition.

To prevent and reverse iron-deficiency anemia, an effort should be made to supply the child with iron-rich foods that she finds appealing. Try dried apricots, raisins, prunes, bananas, egg yolks, blackstrap molasses, wheat germ, sunflower and sesame seeds, beans, peas, whole grains, soybeans, chemical-free red meat, spinach, carrots, and beets. The diet should include plenty of protein and green vegetables. Some health food stores sell iron tonics made from herbs. As mentioned above, iron supplements can be dangerously toxic, even fatal in an overdose; if they must be used, they should never be left within a child's reach.

Good sources of folic acid are leafy green vegetables, broccoli, oranges, and cantaloupe. Vitamin B_{12} is found in fish, poultry, and meat. Nonmeat food sources include eggs, dairy products, tempeh (a food made from soybeans), peanuts, and Concord grapes. Copper is found in nuts, seafood, molasses, and legumes.

Supplements that can help the body use iron efficiently include balanced B-complex including pantothenic acid and B_{12}, vitamins C and E, kelp tablets, and bone meal. Except in small doses (as found in a children's multiple vitamin-mineral tablet) nutrients such as copper and cobalt should come from food, not supplements.

HERB TEAS. Raspberry leaf, red clover, rose hip, parsley, comfrey, alfalfa, nettle, dandelion, fenugreek, yellow dock root.

ACUPRESSURE AND MASSAGE. Rub firmly with the fingertips all along the sternum (breastbone), concentrating on tender points.

APPENDICITIS

The appendix is a short, finger-shaped, blind tube attached to the cecum, the bulge near the beginning of the large intestine. Until fairly recently, many doctors considered the appendix a purposeless vestigial organ, but it is now known to contain functional lymphatic tissue and to contribute to the digestive system's immune function. Because of its structure, the appendix cannot drain itself of infected matter if it becomes inflamed. The cause of appendicitis does not seem to be specific, but diets relying heavily on low-fiber foods may be partly to blame; appendicitis is very rare among people whose diets are high in unrefined foods.

The symptoms of appendicitis are constant pain and tenderness in the abdomen, with or without fever. A child may complain of pain first in the center, around the belly button, and later have the pain move toward the lower right. A very small child may not be able to tell you where the pain is, but he will be quite distressed and his abdomen very sensitive to touch. In appendicitis, the pain is not made better by passing gas or having a bowel movement. There is often some fever but it is not necessarily high, and there may be nausea and loss of appetite. The child may lie with his right leg bent, and may find it hard to stand on only the right leg and support the weight of his body.

It is rare for appendicitis to occur in a child under age five, but most cases do occur in people under thirty. There seems to be some familial predisposition for appendicitis, so if other members of the family have had it, the possibility should be especially considered when a child is distressed with abdominal pain.

WHAT A PHYSICIAN MAY DO

A doctor will examine the child's abdomen, ask questions about the pain location and other symptoms, take a blood sample to look for increased white blood cells (which indicate infection), and check for fever. Because appendicitis can occur without a significant rise in temperature or in white blood count, whether surgery is indicated is sometimes a difficult decision for a doctor to make.

If the decision is made to remove the appendix, the operation (appendectomy) is usually performed right away. Should an abscess be found on the appendix, it has to be drained before removal, and antibiotic injections given to prevent peritonitis (see below).

WHAT YOU CAN DO AT HOME

PRACTICAL MEASURES. If a child has a serious case of appendicitis, surgery may be the best solution. If the appendix is badly inflamed or gangrenous and you wait too long, it may burst and cause peritonitis. Peritonitis is an inflammation of the membranous sac that surrounds the abdominal organs, usually caused by the spread of infected matter. It is extremely dangerous and sometimes fatal. Do not give an enema or laxative if appendicitis is even slightly suspected.

Appendicitis is not always easy to diagnose, even for a physician. There are, however, some indicators that may help. Very gently touch the child's abdomen all over, to try to find a specific area of pain, or try to get the child to point to it. Flex her right thigh cautiously toward her torso, and see if this causes alarm. Draw an imaginary line between the navel and the bony bump in front of the right hip, then push firmly at its midpoint with your fingertips, quickly pulling your hand away. If this makes the child cry out, she likely has an inflamed appendix. If none of the signs are clear, it is usually safe to wait for several hours (and use gentle home treatments, described below) to see if the pain goes away. If pain remains constant or gets worse, don't wait much longer. Call a doctor for advice.

NUTRITION. Do not give food to a child who seems to have appendicitis.

HERB TEAS. Echinacea, calendula.

HOMEOPATHIC REMEDIES.

Arsenicum album. Violent abdominal distress, worse after midnight; child may be fearful, restless though exhausted, chilly.

Belladonna. Onset of pain is sudden and accompanied by fever, worse from gentle pressure and jarring; child may be flushed, with stupor or pounding pulse.

Bryonia. Pain is worse on breathing, coughing, or the slightest motion; child may be irritable, dizzy on sitting up, dry-mouthed, thirsty, and worse from warmth.

Colocynthis. Cramping, grinding pains, better from hard pressure or doubling up, and from warmth; child may have been angry or outraged before pains began.

Dioscorea. Cutting pains radiating to the back, chest, arms; pain is better from standing, moving around, or bending backwards; worse from lying down or doubling up.

Mercurius corrosivus. Bloated abdomen with a bruised feeling, especially in the right lower section, and painful urging in the rectum; worse at night and from touch.

Phosphorus. Cutting pains with an empty sensation in the abdomen; the child is thirsty, but later nauseous as water warms in the stomach; child is fearful, imaginative.

Rhus toxicodendron. Violent pain that requires the child to walk bent over; pains are relieved by lying on abdomen; better from motion and warmth; worse lying on back or right side, and at night.

Silicea. Hard, bloated abdomen, with painful cold feeling; child may be a "refined," fastidious type, easily tired, with a tendency to headaches and big bowel movements.

ACUPRESSURE AND MASSAGE. These points may be found and pressed or rubbed for several minutes to help the body fight the infection. They are *not* substitutes for medical care.

SP 6: A tender point three of the child's finger-breadths above the inner anklebone.

ST 36: A tender point next to the side of the big bump at the top of the shin.

P 6: A point in the mid-forearm, three of the child's finger-breadths above the palm-side wrist-crease.

BL 25: Points in the muscles just to the sides of the lowest two vertebrae.

ASTHMA

Asthma is a condition of difficult breathing that usually occurs in children who are highly allergic or under a great deal of emotional stress. It consists of attacks during which the muscular tubes of the lungs' smaller air passages go into spasm, the mucous membranes become swollen, and mucus is secreted in large amounts. During an attack—which may last for minutes, hours, or even days—the child wheezes and often feels panicked or alarmed. He may be able to quickly take in air, but finds it almost impossible to exhale. (The word *asthma,* in Greek, means "panting.") He usually needs to sit up to help the air get through, and his face may become red from the effort, or sometimes pale or even bluish from lack of oxygen (a danger sign). At the end of an attack, the child may cough violently, bringing up sticky mucus, after which breathing becomes easier.

Because it is thought to be primarily an allergic disorder compounded by emotional stress, the best long-term treatment for asthma is to find out what triggers the attack and to keep the child from being exposed to it, as well as helping to diminish allergic response by building up the child's general health and resistance. (See ALLERGIES.) Some experts believe that children who have had their tonsils and adenoids taken out, and have thus been deprived of lymphatic tissues designed to defend against infection and allergens, are likely to go on to have asthma.

Asthma is very intense and often frightening, both for the child and his family, although it is unlikely that a simple asthma attack that is uncomplicated by infection will be life-threatening. *Any* attack of wheezing, however, is potentially serious—

especially if the child has never had such an attack before. It is possible that the child has inhaled a foreign object that must be removed immediately (see the chapter on Emergencies in Part One) or has a severe respiratory infection that needs a doctor's care. If the attack is very severe—that is, if it seems that the child is really not getting enough air, has blue discoloration in the face or nailbeds, is very confused, distressed, or lethargic—and home care measures (below) do not seem to help significantly, it is best to get help from a doctor right away.

WHAT A PHYSICIAN MAY DO

During an acute asthma attack, a doctor will listen to the child's lungs and heart, then—if the troubled breathing seems severe—give a shot of epinephrine (adrenaline) or a dose of theophylline. These medications relax the muscles in the bronchial tubes and make more room in the passages so the child can breathe. Side effects may be a "hyper" feeling, rapid heartbeat, sleeplessness, and shakiness. Some doctors will want the child to continue to take theophylline for a week or more following an attack. Others will prescribe corticosteroid drugs, given orally or in an aerosol inhaler. The dosage of these medications must be watched very carefully.

If a doctor wants to use long-term medication, be sure to find out how it works and what its side effects might be. Remember that drugs do not remove the allergies or emotional stresses that trigger the attacks, nor do they strengthen and balance the child's constitution. While bringing temporary relief, they can cause other extremely serious problems. Corticosteroids have been known to disrupt endocrine balance and damage children's growth, metabolism, muscular and nervous function, and appearance. Aerosol medications are probably the safest and most effective of any of the asthma-related drugs, as they don't get in the bloodstream and the amount administered is regulated more carefully than it used to be in the past.

Some physicians use nutrition, homeopathy, manipulations, acupuncture, herbs, and other natural remedies to help correct asthmatic conditions. If your child has asthma, it is worth your while to look for a holistic program by which to lessen or prevent attacks and reduce the need for hospital care or medications.

WHAT YOU CAN DO AT HOME

PRACTICAL MEASURES. During an acute attack, find out in what position it is easiest for the child to breathe, and place pillows so it is easier for him to relax.

Try to have the child drink a lot of water, juice, or herb teas to reduce the moisture lost by panting and sweating and to loosen the bronchial secretions. Some cases have been relieved by adding an infusion of thyme (three ounces of leaves, steeped in a pint of boiling water) to the bathwater. Thyme or eucalyptus (oil or leaves) may be added to a vaporizer or humidifier.

Stepping out into the fresh air or taking a ride in the car often helps a child to breathe and to relax. (Keep in mind that, if pollution levels are high in your area, the air is not fresh!)

Breathing exercises: Have the child imagine his abdomen and chest as a huge balloon that he will fill with air—slowly, starting from the bottom—by inhaling. Now have him empty it slowly, keeping his mouth tight and round as though whistling. Calm, confident, quiet coaching will help him do this slowly, without panic. This exercise should be done daily, as well as during episodes of asthma.

PREVENTIVE MEASURES.

- Do not allow smoking in the house. Turn off central heating in the asthmatic child's bedroom to avoid circulating allergenic particles. (See ALLERGIES.)
- Encourage the child to take up an active sport to strengthen and exercise the lungs; swimming is ideal if he does not react to chlorine or have frequent colds.
- Talk to your child and make him feel free to express his opinions and emotions. Be involved in his life, but not in a suffocating way; be sure he can "breathe."

NUTRITION. Strengthen the child's resistance with good nutrition. The diet should consist of fresh, unrefined foods, plenty of fruits and vegetables, and good-quality protein. Eating raw garlic and thyme every day (a good way to get them down is in salad dressing) seems to help some children. Onions, mustard, horseradish, and chili peppers may also help, if the child will eat them. Supplements of vitamins C and E and manganese are helpful. (See also ALLERGIES.) During attacks or threatened attacks, give 100–250 mg of vitamin C every few hours.

HERB TEAS. During an attack: ephedra (Mormon tea), coltsfoot, yerba santé, wild cherry bark, ginger root. Daily: peppermint, red clover, comfrey, nettle, parsley, thyme.

HOMEOPATHIC REMEDIES. The following remedies are useful in acute attacks. A child with recurrent asthma should receive constitutional treatment from a trained homeopathic practitioner. See also COUGHS for other remedies.

Arsenicum album. Dry, wheezing asthma ending with white, frothy sputum; attacks begin near or after midnight; child is chilly or has hot head and cold extremities, is oversensitive to smells, fearful, restless but exhausted, and uneasy lying down.

Antimonium tartaricum. Mucus in the chest sounds wet, bubbly, frothy; child coughs and gapes, has a rapid pulse, feels dizzy; feels better lying on the right side, sitting up, and from spitting and burping.

Chamomilla. Dry, tickling cough, rattling mucus, worse with wind and at night; child is very agitated, irritable, oversensitive, hot; anger may precipitate an attack.

Ipecacuanha. Wheezing begins abruptly with heaviness in the chest; there is profuse mucus that can't be coughed up; long spasms of coughing may end in vomiting.

Nux vomica. Constriction in the chest, worse in the morning, after eating, or following an upset stomach; better in the evening or damp weather; child may be pushy or irritable.

Pulsatilla. Wheezing usually starts in the evening; is especially bad in a warm or stuffy room and is much better from fresh air; child may be tearful and sweet, wanting to be held and comforted.

ACUPRESSURE AND MASSAGE.

GB 20: A tender point in the muscles just below the base of the skull, midway between the central bump on the lower back of the head and the ear tip.

BL 2: A point just below the bony ridge of the eyebrow, at the end near the nose.

CV 22: A point in the notch at the base of the throat, just above the breastbone.

LU 1: A tender point in the indentation below the shoulder end of the collarbone.

LI 4: The point at the end of the crease between the thumb and index finger, massage the thumb webs.

LI 11: A tender point at the thumb-side end of the elbow-crease when the arm is bent.

- With your right hand, massage the muscles on both sides of the spine from the nape of the neck to the bottom of the rib cage; at the same time, use your left hand to gently rub the rib-heads (the row of tender bumps on each side of the sternum).
- Deep massage of the upper back and shoulders helps some children. A long backrub or footrub, along with a story read aloud, may distract and calm them.

Bedwetting

Bedwetting is a normal part of life for very small children. Just as it takes time for a waking child to be toilet trained, it takes time for the child's nervous system to learn to control the bladder during sleep. Bedwetting, up to the age of six, should not arouse much concern unless there is some indication that the cause is emotional, or that there is a problem in the urinary tract or spinal column (under which circumstances the child would probably have difficulty with bladder control in the daytime as well as during sleep).

Even up to the age of ten or twelve, an occasional episode of bedwetting should not be alarming, especially with a nervous or excitable child. When it happens regularly to children this old, however, other reasons should be considered, such as allergies, emotional difficulties (sometimes an anxious child who feels the need for more attention will "regress"), episodes of low blood sugar, urinary tract infections, spinal problems, and structural problems in kidneys or bladder.

WHAT A PHYSICIAN MAY DO

A doctor will probably ask how often the bedwetting happens, at what time of night, and under what circumstances. If a physical defect is suspected, such as malfunctioning or malformation of the kidneys, ureters, bladder, or urethra, a urine sample may be taken and analyzed, and an examination of the urinary and genital structures may be performed. If the doctor wants X-ray studies of the kidney and bladder, you should find out exactly why he thinks they are necessary, and get a second and perhaps third opinion. X rays are always hazardous, and seldom necessary for this sort of diagnosis.

Some doctors prescribe drugs (such as imipramine, Dilantin, or dextroamphetamine) to control bedwetting. Whether these medications work is debatable—and even if a child taking them wets the bed less, this is a drug-induced change in symptoms, not an improvement in bladder control. Such medications may have dangerous side effects: imipramine can cause convulsions, digestive disorders, collapse, and even death. Most parents would choose the frequent inconvenience of a wet bed over taking such a risk.

Most doctors do not prescribe drugs and approach the bedwetting problem moderately, with recommendations similar to those below. If you feel the need to work on this with a health care professional, be sure it is a person with whom the child can be comfortable. If the child feels humiliated, pressured, or self-conscious, the problem may be prolonged.

WHAT YOU CAN DO AT HOME

PRACTICAL MEASURES. Try not to let a wet bed seem like a big deal. Be ready with dry pajamas and easily changed bedding so the child (and you) can get back to sleep as soon as possible. Keep pads or rubber sheets on the mattress to protect it. Don't let the child feel that you are disgusted or irritated; it isn't much fun to get up in the night to change sheets and clothes, but wetting the bed is not a voluntary act, and anxiety is likely to make it happen more often.

It may help a little to have the child eat fruit instead of drinking fluids when he's thirsty in the evening, and to remind him to empty his bladder just before bedtime—although it is acquiring unconscious control of the bladder that really counts, regardless of how full it is.

Candy or desserts eaten in the evening increase the likelihood of a wet bed: concentrated sweets cause the blood sugar to rise at first, then, as the body tries to compensate for the surfeit of sugar, to drop very low; this low blood-sugar level deprives the nervous system of the fuel (glucose) it needs to function, and the nerve centers for unconscious bladder control may miss some messages. Pressures, fears, and worries during the day may also cause a drop in blood sugar after the child has fallen asleep.

Exercises in bladder control may be useful. During the day, the child should be encouraged to drink lots of water, juice, and teas and, when she feels a full bladder, to "hold it" as long as she can (without embarrassment). While urinating, she should try to stop and start the flow of urine by tightening and relaxing the muscles of the pelvic floor.

Most important in helping a child overcome bedwetting are patience, love, and reassurance. In nearly every case, time eventually takes care of the problem.

NUTRITION. Although celery has diuretic qualities, eating it daily has been of benefit to bedwetters. A handful of raisins before bed has also been helpful. The child should avoid beans, cooked cabbage, or any other foods that seems to cause digestive trouble or gas.

Supplements of B-complex vitamins and magnesium are often effective.

HERB TEAS. These should be drunk earlier in the day, not right before bedtime: cornsilk, cinnamon, fennel, hops, oatstraw, comfrey root, marjoram.

HOMEOPATHIC REMEDIES.

Argentum nitricum. Child wets bed after eating lots of sweets and salt, which are craved; fear of heights and anxiety over minor or imagined things.

Belladonna. Sleep may be restless, and jarring may induce bedwetting; worse after midnight and in changeable weather; child may be strong-willed and nervous.

Causticum. Child wets the bed in early sleep, and may even wet her pants during the day, when sneezing, laughing, or after some excitement; bedwetting more frequent in cold or rainy weather.

Cina. Child is peevish, dissatisfied, does not like to be looked at or touched; may have worms; grinds his teeth, picks his nose.

Equiseteum. Frequent wetting without a clear cause; pressure or slight pain in the bladder not relieved by urinating; child wets bed during nightmares or other dreams.

Kreosotum. Child dreams of urinating and wets the bed, usually during the first part of the night; sleeps very deeply and is hard to wake.

Lycopodium. Lots of urine is passed, making the skin red or irritated; gas or bloating, especially in late afternoon and evening; child may be insecure.

Phosphorus. Lots of colorless urine; and child is very affectionate, imaginative and bright; is afraid of the dark, of ghosts, and of being alone; craves ice cream and salt.

Pulsatilla. For sweet, weepy children who sleep with hands above the head; worse in a warm or stuffy room and after rich food; urine may have an offensive smell.

Sepia. Wets in the first hours of sleep; worse in cold weather; child may fear ghosts and thunder, and feel better after exercise.

ACUPRESSURE AND MASSAGE.

· Rub the top two little-finger creases, on the palm side, for about one minute each.

KI 3: The tender point just behind the upper rear aspect of the inner anklebone.

GV 20: The tender point (a slightly soft spot) at the very top of the head.

BITES (Animal or Human)

Any animal bite, whether a stallion's chomp, a cat-tooth puncture, a scratch from a puppy's jaw, or a bite from a little brother, should be cared for right away. The mammals that most frequently bite children are dogs, cats, and other children—but geese, ponies, mice, guinea pigs, goats, sheep, and cattle bite, too. The type of care needed will depend upon the depth and size of the wound, how dirty it is, and on what area of the body it has been inflicted. If the bite is not large and is not on the face or some delicate tissue, and if the animal is your pet or a neighbor's and is known not to be diseased, there is little cause to worry, as long as the wound is thoroughly cleaned. If the owner is unknown, or if the animal was acting strangely, attacked unprovoked, or is wild—a skunk, possum, raccoon, fox, or bat, for example—the possibility of rabies has to be considered. (See RABIES.) If the bite makes a puncture that does not bleed enough to carry infective material out of the wound, steps should be taken to prevent tetanus. (See PUNCTURE WOUNDS.)

A bite on the face, even a moderate one, should be seen by a doctor, to ensure safe healing without disfigurement.

WHAT A PHYSICIAN MAY DO

A doctor will examine, clean, and disinfect the wound, then close the wound edges with stitches or special bandaging, if necessary. Treatment may be begun for rabies or tetanus if there seems to be danger of these. Some doctors are inclined to give tetanus shots more often than they are truly indicated (some physicians give a booster shot any time the skin is broken, whereas the organisms responsible for tetanus require a puncture wound, or a wound in which dirt in the damaged tissue is sealed off from air, to produce the disease). See Part Two chapter on Immunizations.

WHAT YOU CAN DO AT HOME

To clean a puncture wound, the tissue around the hole should be pressed carefully but firmly to make it bleed. Bleeding is likely to wash out the deeper parts of the puncture and decrease the possibility of tetanus.

For a tear, cut, or scratch, first hold the wounded areas under cold running water, then wash it thoroughly with soap and water, followed by a disinfectant such as tincture of calendula, hypericum, or echinacea (diluted 5:1 with water), or hydrogen peroxide. Tinctures of ledum or hypericum are good for puncture wounds.

A tobacco poultice can draw infectious material out of a puncture wound. Dampen a large pinch of pouch tobacco (or the contents of a cigarette) and place it on the puncture for fifteen minutes.

For nutrition, homeopathic remedies, and acupressure points see INFECTIONS.

BEES, YELLOWJACKETS, WASPS, and HORNETS

Most of these stings are instantly painful and produce pink, swollen areas that last a few hours or days, go on to itch, and are usually not too serious. Some people, however, react allergically to the venom in a sting and may go into shock, or even die. Signs of such reaction are very rapid and severe swelling at the site of the bite, wheezing, a sensation of swelling or blockage in the mouth and throat, fainting, confusion, hives or a skin rash, and abdominal pain. If any of these symptoms is evident or has occurred with prior stings, get medical help immediately. Some allergic persons carry "bee-sting" kits, containing a small syringe of epinephrine (adrenaline). In the case of such reaction, the epinephrine should be administered right away—on the way to the doctor if possible.

WHAT A PHYSICIAN MAY DO

Antihistamines or analgesic corticosteroid lotion medications may be given for nonemergency stings. If a sting causes an extreme allergic reaction, a doctor will give a shot of epinephrine. If the child's throat is so swollen that she cannot breathe, a tracheotomy (an emergency operation that involves cutting an artificial opening in the swollen airways) may be performed. CPR will be given if breathing or heartbeat has stopped. (See Emergencies chapter in Part Two.)

WHAT YOU CAN DO AT HOME

If the stinger is still in the skin, try to remove it by brushing or scraping it away instead of pulling, which may cause more venom to be released. To relieve pain and reduce swelling, place ice on the area, alternately applying any of the following: ledum tincture (diluted 5:1), vitamin E oil, aloe vera gel; vinegar, lemon, or lime juice (for wasp and hornet stings); or a paste of baking soda and water (for honeybee stings). If there are multiple stings and the child seems very ill or shows signs of allergic reaction (see above, and ALLERGIES), get medical help immediately.

HOMEOPATHIC REMEDIES.

Apis mellifica. Much pink swelling, heat, and stinging pain; worse from heat and touch.

Ledum palustre. Swelling extends far around the bite; stung area may feel cold or numb.

Crotalus horridus. Much pain, sickness, and severe swelling that comes on quickly after the bite. (If this remedy is indicated, get medical help right away.)

Carbolicum acidum. Child's face becomes dark or red, and pale around the mouth; there is stupor and difficulty breathing, even paralysis, but sense of smell may be heightened. (If this remedy is indicated, the condition is serious; get medical help right away.)

Note: Homeopathic *Apis mellifica* and *Carbolicum acidum* given during cases of allergic shock have been known to save lives. If a family member has ever had an extreme reaction to stings or bites, these remedies should be kept in the car or carried by that person in a first-aid kit.

SPIDER BITES

Most spider bites, if examined closely, show two punctures in the middle of a welt. The bites are often more tender and longer-lasting than those of fleas or mosquitoes. If the bite is on the face or leads to serious illness, medical help should be sought right away. Common poisonous spiders in North America include:

· The *black widow,* a shiny black spider with a red hourglass mark on its abdomen. This spider's bite is not very painful at first, but may be followed within ten minutes to an hour by intense pain, muscle cramping (of the abdomen, shoulders, chest, or back) nausea, headache, sweating, and shaking.

· The *brown recluse* or violin spider, a brown spider with a dark violin-shaped mark on its back. This spider's bite can also go un-noticed for an hour or more. It then begins to hurt, and creates a "bulls-eye" ulcer or blood blister that can continue over weeks to increase in size and damage underlying tissues.

Even if you haven't found the spider, if a child has any of these symptoms, see a doctor right away.

WHAT A PHYSICIAN MAY DO

For a black widow bite, the doctor may admit the child to the hospital, where antivenin will be given after a skin test to check for allergic reaction. Calcium gluconate solution may be given intravenously to control the muscle pain and spasm. Vital signs will be checked frequently for the first day after the bite.

For a new brown recluse bite, a doctor may choose to excise (cut out) the injured area to stop the spreading of the ulcer. Corticosteroid drugs may be given if the bite occurred within the previous forty-eight hours. The ulcers are cleaned with hydrogen peroxide or other disinfectants, the damaged tissues cut or scraped away, and antibiotic ointments given to apply at home.

WHAT YOU CAN DO AT HOME

Putting ice on the bite may temporarily slow the swelling and spread of venom. If the biting spider is known to be poisonous (see above), or the reaction to the bite is severe, get to a doctor right away. The child's life may be in danger. You can still use natural therapies en route—certainly put ice on the area—but don't wait too long.

If the offending spider was not a dangerous one, apply ice to the bite, alternating with ledum or hypericum tincture (diluted 5:1) or vitamin E oil. Vitamin C and calcium, taken internally, may be helpful.

For homeopathic remedies, see BEES etc. above.

Other types of insect bites, unless a child is allergic to them or the lesions become badly infected from scratching, usually do not require a doctor's care.

FLEAS

Fleas often give multiple bites, which usually do no more than itch, although the reactions vary from person to person and with the number of bites. Fleas can occasionally cause hives by means of a protein they carry, even without biting.

To prevent fleabites, the house should be vacuumed frequently and all bedding kept clean and aired. Chemical flea collars, powders, soaps, and sprays for use on animals should not be used near children (or adults); they are very toxic. Natural flea powders or sprays containing *pyrethrins* (made from pyrethrum flowers) are deadly to fleas and other insects and fish, but not to mammals, although some people are allergic to them. Citronella, eucalyptus, cedar, bay, and pennyroyal oils sprinkled on bedding or dabbed on the skin, and eating raw garlic every day, may help keep fleas from biting. Bites may be soothed with aloe vera juice, lemon juice, or vitamin E oil. Extra vitamin C taken internally will lessen itching.

LICE

Lice leave tiny, pinpoint-sized red sores at the base of hairs, and are usually detected by the presence of nits (egg clusters that look like tiny white grains of rice adhering to hair strands). Outbreaks of lice occur frequently, even in the cleanest schools and daycare centers. If you hear of an outbreak that might have affected your child, search for nits in the hair of all family members. If you find any, have everyone bathe thoroughly, and treat the hair and scalp.

A natural remedy for lice can be made by combining a tea-spoonful each of pennyroyal, eucalyptus, and rosemary oils with five to six tablespoons of olive oil. Wash the child's hair in water as hot as she can stand, and dry it with a towel. Test the oil mixture on your skin, and also test a very small part of the child's scalp, to be sure it doesn't burn. (It will tingle but shouldn't hurt. If it does, add more olive oil.) Apply the oil to her hair and scalp. The smell will be very strong, so tell her what to expect. Comb the oil through her hair; comb out and dispose of any nits. Wrap the child's head in a towel or washable cloth and leave the oil on all night. The next day, shampoo her hair thoroughly (more than once, if necessary). If lice reappear, repeat this procedure.

Lotions of benzyl benzoate or gamma benzene hexachloride (Kwell, Nix, and RID are some brand names) are often used to kill lice. These are toxic, so if you use them, read all instructions and warnings first; if there is any sign of swelling, skin irritation, breathing difficulty, or other side effects, wash the child's hair and scalp thoroughly and call a doctor for advice. Before using these medications, give the child extra vitamin C to help combat toxicity.

Don't forget to boil, steam-clean, or dry-clean all linens and clothing, pillows, hats, brushes, and combs that might have been exposed. If such things are too hard to sterilize, wrap them in plastic and place them in a deep freeze for several weeks, or throw them away. Lice can recur if not eradicated thoroughly.

MOSQUITO BITES

Prevention of bites is the best course to take if mosquitoes are swarming about. Some experts recommend that, if you must mingle with these shrill and irritating insects, you should take a teaspoonful of brewer's yeast in water every hour; they claim the mosquitoes dislike the smell and taste (although children usually dislike it as well). Eating raw garlic is also said to dissuade mosquitoes from biting. Citronella and eucalyptus oils are natural repellents. Cool damp cloths applied to the bites, aloe vera juice (fresh from a plant), lemon juice, or vitamin E oil may calm the itching. Extra vitamin C will help reduce swelling and itching.

TICKS

After walking through thick underbrush, all hikers should be checked for ticks. When a tick has moved in, it may not feel like much, but its fat little reddish-gray body can be seen protruding from the person's skin while the head is inside, drinking blood. To make the tick let go, dab its protruding body with alcohol, acetone, kerosene, or oil, or touch it with a heated paper clip. If it does not back out, grasping the body and twisting it counterclockwise may make it release its grip. If the body comes off and the head remains in the flesh, soak the area gently with warm water several times a day until the tick's head comes out and the tissues heal. Use calendula, echinacea, or ledum tinctures (diluted 5:1) as disinfectant. Give extra vitamin C to help fight infection. Ticks can carry diseases, such as Lyme disease, various fevers, and tick paralysis, though these are not common. If any strange symptoms—infection around the bite, blistering, fever, flulike illness, headache, stiff neck, swollen joints, or paralysis—occur within a few weeks after a tick bite, see a doctor. (Lyme disease is treated with antibiotics.)

CHIGGERS

Chiggers are tiny red itching sores that contain mite larvae. When these sores are scratched, the larval sac is broken and more of the itch-causing chemical is released. Avoiding the insects' haunts is the best prevention for bites (they are usually found in the Southern part of the United States), but if you are around their habitat, wear sturdy, tucked-in clothing. Insect repellents (natural ones are citronella, cedar, and eucalyptus oil) may keep the mites away, and bathing right after exposure can reduce the chance of itchy infestation. Over-the-counter lotions of benzyl benzoate or GBH may kill the larvae, but since the itch is from a chemical the bugs release inside your skin, once it starts it will go on awhile. Extra vitamin C and ice applications may help relieve itching.

SCABIES

Scabies usually shows up in skin creases such as armpits, groin, behind the knees, inside elbows, and between fingers. Trails or burrowing tracks are seen on the skin, which reddens, swells, or blisters. You can treat scabies yourself, but if the home remedies are slow to work, consulting a health care professional is not a bad idea, because scabies is desperately uncomfortable and very contagious. The nonnatural remedy, a 25 percent solution of benzyl benzoate, can be obtained from a pharmacy without a prescription;

directions will say to apply it to every part of the body except the orifices and face. Natural remedies used for treating scabies include juniper berry tea: steep a tablespoonful of berries in a pint of boiling water. Apply the cooled tea to the skin, then drink the rest throughout the day, for as long as the itching lasts. Or apply sulphur powder mixed with alcohol to the itching parts, or wash the scabies tracks with tincture of green soap. To diminish the itching, some people prefer long, hot soaks, and others cool compresses. Use whichever makes your child feel the best. All affected clothes and bedding should be thoroughly washed and dried in a hot drier, or boiled, or thrown away.

HOMEOPATHIC REMEDIES.
> *Mercurius vivus.* Given on the first day, followed the next day by *Sulphur.* A homeopathic physician may give a more specific prescription, according to the individual patient's needs.

SNAKEBITE

Bites from poisonous snakes are always emergencies. Symptoms include a double puncture mark surrounded by swelling and bruising. The bite does not always hurt. The child may sweat, have chills, be nauseous, vomit or cough up blood, or have convulsions. When death occurs from snakebite, it is often from shock or respiratory distress. The size of the child and the area of the body bitten, how much venom was injected, the kind of snake, and how quickly the bite is treated are all factors in how serious a snakebite is, but no chances should be taken; medical help should be found immediately. Unfortunately, most snakebites occur some distance from an emergency room. While traveling (or waiting) for medical help, the child should be calmed and comforted and kept as still as possible; the wound can be washed with cool water, and the bitten area placed in a position lower than the heart. If medical help is more than half an hour away, the body part should also be firmly wrapped with a wide strip of cloth, as close as possible to the bite (the band placed on the side that is nearer to the heart), to slow the spread of the venom. Check this often; if swelling has made the band too tight, loosen it. Homeopathic remedies listed above (see BEES etc.) may help with snakebite. If you use them, still *do not* neglect to see a physician.

BLEEDING

BLEEDING FROM WOUNDS

If the blood is oozing slowly, not dripping or spurting, the wound is probably not dangerous. If, however, it seems that a great deal of blood is being lost, immediate attempts should be made to slow it. Remember that a child is smaller than an adult, thus cannot afford to lose as much blood.

Find the cleanest available cloth (if there is no clean cloth, use your fingers) and apply direct pressure to the wound. If it is possible to raise the injured part to a level higher than the head and heart, this may help slow the bleeding. If blood is spurting out, try to press the wound (and thereby the opened blood vessel) against the underlying bone. If the cut is in the armpit or groin where bones are not accessible, wad up the cleanest cloth you can find and press it against the wound as hard as you can. Keep the pressure on, and send for help immediately. If there is no one around to assist you, carry the child only if you are able to stop the bleeding by pressure while you do. If this is not possible, bind an object over the wound that is heavy enough to stop the bleeding by pressure, and leave the child in a sheltered place while you go for help.

NATURAL REMEDIES. A tincture or tea of the herb shepherd's purse, taken internally, can help stop bleeding. Vitamin C may help.

To help ensure that a child's blood will clot correctly should he receive an injury, his daily diet should include foods rich in vitamin K: alfalfa sprouts, green leafy vegetables, kelp, egg yolks and soybeans are good sources. Aspirin and antibiotics can work against vitamin K in the body. Lactobacillus-cultured milk products such as yogurt and kefir help support the benign intestinal bacteria that produce vitamin K.

HOMEOPATHIC REMEDIES. (If the child seems disoriented or unconscious, the remedy pellet should be crushed or dissolved in water and touched to the mucous membrane inside the mouth, to avoid aspiration or choking.)

Arnica montana. Wound is from a blow or fall, or child has shock symptoms.

Ipecacuanha. Profuse gushing or spurting bleeding; child may feel nauseous, clammy, weak.

Phosphorus. Small wounds that bleed a lot; child may show small red pinpoints of bleeding under the skin.

BLEEDING FROM HEAD WOUNDS

Head wounds tend to bleed profusely even when the injury is minor, because the heart sends an abundance of blood to the head to keep the brain supplied with oxygen, and the tissues of the scalp, face, eyes, nose, mouth, and gums are rich with blood vessels. If the wound has come from a blow or fall, check for concussion or skull fracture; these may be emergencies, and the child should see a doctor. (See HEAD INJURIES.) Otherwise, apply direct pressure over the wound with a clean cloth or bandage until the bleeding is controlled.

INTERNAL BLEEDING

If, after a fall or hard blow to the abdomen or head, a child's pulse is very slow, very rapid, or irregular, this may be a sign of internal bleeding. The child may seem disoriented or the muscles of her abdomen may become rigid. Call a doctor right away. A doctor should also be consulted if a child is coughing up blood, or if bowel movements are black or very dark, which may be a sign of bleeding in the digestive tract.

RECTAL BLEEDING

If bright red blood comes out of a child's rectum, there has probably been a slight tear in a lower part of the digestive tract; this is often caused by constipation, or, sometimes—with young, experimentally inclined children—foreign objects. (See CONSTIPATION and FOREIGN OBJECTS.)

VAGINAL BLEEDING

During the first two weeks of life, some baby girls bleed a little from the vagina because of hormones received while they shared the mother's blood before birth.

Menstrual periods that are considered normal may occur as early as age eight or ten, depending upon the child. If a girl begins to bleed from her vagina at this age, however, a doctor's opinion should be sought—both for the sake of ruling out more serious problems and to reassure the child, who may be frightened. (See MENSTRUAL PROBLEMS.)

BLISTERS

Blisters are small areas in which fluid has collected under the caused by friction (new shoes that rub, zealous swinging on the monkey-bars), or may appear as a result of burns, sunburn, chilblains, poison oak or ivy, insect bites, ringworm, impetigo, scabies, or chicken pox. Usually the cause is obvious. (See appropriate sections for care of specific conditions.) If red streaks begin to extend from a broken blister, the lymph vessels in the area are becoming inflamed; this could be a signal of spreading infection and may be serious.

WHAT A PHYSICIAN MAY DO

Special protective padding may be applied if blisters are in areas that get a lot of friction. A doctor will usually give antibiotics if lymphangitis, infection, or fever is present. (Natural remedies often work very well in such situations.)

WHAT YOU CAN DO AT HOME

PRACTICAL MEASURES. Protect blisters so they don't get dirty or infected. If possible, do not drain, prick, or break them—the fluid will be reabsorbed by the body eventually, and unbroken skin is a good protection against infection. If the pressure is really bothersome, or you think that the child is likely to burst the blister anyway, an adult should clean and drain it. The area should first be disinfected, then a needle (sterilized by holding the pointed half in a flame) should be inserted near the edge, with great care being taken not to poke the tender nearby tissue; the liquid may then be pressed out. If a blister has been drained or burst, encourage the child not to peel the skin off, as the tissue will be raw and sore underneath and the flap of skin can protect it.

Blisters may be bandaged lightly to keep them clean, but be sure the air can reach them. If the blister is on the sole of the foot or some other place where pressure can't be avoided, a ring of dry cotton held on by gauze and tape, or a circle of mole-foam applied around the circumference of the blister, can save it from further insult. If blisters were caused by shoes, make sure the child wears other shoes during healing; the offending shoes should be worn only for short periods later, until they're broken in. Make sure a child with blisters on his feet wears white cotton socks; many dyes are toxic and can cause serious complications if they enter the lymph system or bloodstream.

NATURAL APPLICATIONS. If red streaks or painful inflammation are present, trouble can often be allayed by applying a potato poultice. Wash and peel a healthy raw potato and grate it. Lay a mound of grated potato against the blister, cover it with a clean damp cloth, and leave it on for at least twenty minutes. Tinctures of calendula, echinacea, or goldenseal diluted 5:1 with water may be applied as disinfectants. A mixture of equal parts of powdered slippery-elm bark and powdered comfrey root may be sprinkled on a raw or open blister to form a soothing and protective scab.

For nutrition, herb teas, and homeopathic remedies, see INFECTIONS.

BOILS (Abscesses, Carbuncles)

A boil is a red, hard, tender, infected pocket or lump in skin and underlying tissue, caused by lowered resistance to the staphylococcus bacteria that are normally present on healthy skin. Lowered resistance to infection is often caused by poor nutrition, emotional stress, overwork, lack of sleep, or allergy. Boils usually contain pus, although it may be out of sight below the surface. They can be distinguished from simple pimples by their size, depth, amount of soreness, hardness, and duration. If the child has quite a number of boils, on the face or in the nose, on parts of the body that are difficult to keep clean (ears, anus, armpits), in pressure areas (knees or buttocks), or if a boil is accompanied by fever, swollen lymph nodes, or red streaks into adjacent tissues, it may be best to see a doctor.

WHAT A PHYSICIAN MAY DO
A doctor will examine the boil for size and seriousness, and check for undetected wounds, splinters, or foreign bodies. He may ask questions about the child's overall health, nutrition, and resistance to infection. If he decides that the boil should be lanced, he will make a small incision with a sterile instrument so the pus can

drain. Many doctors prescribe oral antibiotics or antibiotic ointments to prevent further infection or complications. If the condition does not appear to be severe, parents may prefer to employ
milder, natural remedies.

WHAT YOU CAN DO AT HOME

PRACTICAL MEASURES. Never squeeze a boil, as this may cause
infected matter to be pushed inward, where it may enter the
tissues or bloodstream.

NATURAL APPLICATIONS. Apply a warm, wet cloth to the sore place
several times a day; this will bring more blood and its infection-
fighting elements to the area, and may bring the boil to a head so it
can drain.

Poultices can soothe the area and draw out impurities, thus
keeping the infection from spreading. Place the poultice material
on a thin, untreated, clean cotton cloth, or directly on the skin;
wrap more cloth around it to keep the poultice in place. Leave this
on for half an hour to an hour. Afterwards, gently wash the area
with pure water and cover it with clean gauze. Poultices good for
boils may be made of grated, clean, raw, peeled potato; grated
fresh pumpkin; rolled oats mixed with powdered echinacea powder; or calendula flowers, dampened periodically with tolerably
hot water; cooked onion, cooled to lukewarm; or a cloth soaked
in castor oil.

Once a boil opens and drains, echinacea, goldenseal, or calendula tincture (diluted 1:5 in pure water) may be applied. Ointments made of yellow dock and calendula are also helpful.

Keep all areas of the skin clean by washing with mild soap
and pure water. If the boil does not come to a head or get better in
five days, have a doctor assess it.

NUTRITION. Make sure the child eats nourishing foods, especially
fresh vegetables and fruit, whole grains, and seeds. Have her drink
several glasses of fresh carrot and red beet juices per day. Avoid all
sugar and refined foods and any food to which she might be allergic. This will help strengthen resistance to infection.

A good, balanced vitamin and mineral supplement should be
included in the daily diet. Extra vitamins C, B-complex, A, beta
carotene, and zinc help boils heal.

HERB TEAS. Red clover, echinacea, calendula, comfrey, nettle.

HOMEOPATHIC REMEDIES. If a child has numerous or recurrent boils, constitutional homeopathy from a trained prescriber may help to improve his overall health.

Belladonna. Sore place is red, hot, and throbbing, with little or no pus evident.

Hepar sulphuris calcareum. Very tender, painful boils; there may be sharp pains or a splinterlike sensation; child may be irritable and very sensitive to drafts and cold.

Silicea. Many boils, or boils that form hard lumps and are slow to heal; child may be nervous, headachy, easily fatigued.

Mercurius vivus. Sensitive boils full of pus; pain may be aggravated by warmth; child may drool during sleep, sweat a lot, or have bad breath.

ACUPRESSURE AND MASSAGE.

SP 6: A tender point three of the child's finger-breadths above the inner anklebone.

ST 36: A tender point next to the outer side of the big bump at the top of the shin.

LI 4: The point at the end of the crease between the thumb and index finger.

LI 11: A tender point at the thumb-side end of the elbow-crease when the arm is bent.

BREATH ODORS

Children's breath can smell unpleasant for all sorts of reasons: unbrushed or decaying teeth, unhealthy gums, stomach upsets, bowel disorders, worm infestations, liver malfunction, and infections of the mouth, nose, throat, tonsils, lungs, or sinuses. Bad breath may result from a foreign object lodged in the nose—a predicament quite common among small children. (SEE NOSE CONDITIONS.)

The type of food a child eats contributes to the aroma of his breath. If meat makes up a large part of the diet, putrefactive bacterial products may create an odor as they escape on exhalation from the lungs and digestive tract. The strong smells of garlic and onions linger on the breath, but there's nothing wrong with that.

If the child is otherwise healthy and energetic, the physician of choice is usually a dentist. Only persistent (or strange or awful) bad breath warrants a doctor's attention. If the breath has a sweet or fruity odor (unrelated to recent diet), it may be an indication of diabetes. Sickly sweet breath may signify a liver problem such as hepatitis. Breath that smells like urine may be a sign of a kidney or metabolic problem. If the child is losing weight, urinates very frequently, feels weak or nauseous, or has any other symptoms (swelling, fever, confusion, stupor), see a doctor right away.

WHAT A PHYSICIAN MAY DO

A doctor will give a very ill child a thorough physical examination and do blood and urine tests. Otherwise, she will look for a mouth, throat, or respiratory infection or some disorder in digestion. Antibiotics may be prescribed for infections; laxatives or dietary changes for constipation. If a foreign object is discovered in the nose, the doctor will remove it, probably with forceps, then clear out any putrid matter remaining and deal with infection if one exists.

WHAT YOU CAN DO AT HOME

PRACTICAL MEASURES. If the breath is really malodorous, figure out what's causing it. If the child seems healthy and eats good food, it is likely that the smell is coming from improperly brushed or decaying teeth. It is often hard for small children to brush their teeth thoroughly—and independent ones may vehemently object to being helped. If your child doesn't eat much sugar, and her diet includes raw fruits and vegetables like carrots, celery, and apples every day, her baby teeth will likely be clean enough to last until the permanent teeth come in and she is more adept at brushing them. (See TEETH AND GUMS.)

If the child's breath smells foul from an infection or digestive problem, it is better to correct the cause than simply to cover up the smell with mouthwash. For short-term relief, however, the child can chew on parsley, orange peel, or fennel or anise seed, which make the breath smell nicer.

NUTRITION. An abundance of fresh raw fruit and vegetables should be included in the child's diet. Alfalfa sprouts, tarragon, dill, chickweed, caraway, watercress, and rosemary can be used in salads or soups. Alfalfa tablets, balanced B-complex (especially B_6), vitamin C, zinc, and whey powder can help combat infection, improve digestion, and sweeten the breath.

HERB TEAS. Peppermint, parsley (nice with a bit of cardamom or cloves added), orange peel, ginger root, anise seed, fennel seed, honey and lemon juice.

HOMEOPATHIC REMEDIES. These should not be used symptomatically to control bad breath. If the problem is not corrected by simple hygiene or nutritional measures, the underlying causative condition must be addressed. (See MOUTH AND TONGUE, NOSE CONDITIONS, INDIGESTION AND GAS, CONSTIPATION, ALLERGIES, and other appropriate sections for information on natural ways to deal with these problems.) A trained homeopathic prescriber may be able to help with a constitutional remedy.

BRONCHIOLITIS

This is a virus-related condition seen in infants and toddlers, during which the mucous membranes of the medium-sized breathing tubes (bronchioles) become swollen, reducing the available space for air to pass. Symptoms of bronchiolitis are rapid respiration, a wheezy sound, with difficulty on breathing both in and out. (In CROUP, the trouble is usually worse on breathing in; in ASTHMA, on breathing out. See appropriate sections.)

If there is a very juicy cough, high fever, heaviness or pain in the chest, and the respiratory distress is severe, take the child to a doctor.

WHAT A PHYSICIAN MAY DO
A doctor will take the child's temperature and examine the chest, throat, and neck. The possibility of a more serious bacterial infection, such as pneumonia, will be considered. The doctor may want

to take an X ray of the lungs, but this is rarely necessary, since other symptoms can be used in diagnosis. If the child's breathing is very difficult, drugs such as epinephrine, aminophylline, or theophylline may be prescribed to open the breathing tubes. These may be given by injection, mouth, or rectal suppository.

Sometimes a stay in the hospital is recommended for convenience in giving fluids intravenously, supplying humidified air, and keeping close watch on the child's condition. However, many parents feel they are able to keep close watch on the child themselves. The anxiety the child may feel from being away from home and separated from parents may override the benefits of hospitalization.

WHAT YOU CAN DO AT HOME

PRACTICAL MEASURES. Check to make sure that the breathing trouble is not caused by a foreign object lodged in the throat; children at this age are continually putting odd objects in their mouths. If an object has been inhaled, it must be removed immediately. (See FOREIGN OBJECTS, and the Emergencies chapter in Part Two.)

Watch closely to see that the child's breathing does not become too difficult; infants and toddlers are not always able to say how they feel.

Use a vaporizer or humidifier, or create steam by running a hot shower. Be sure the child gets enough rest and is warm but not uncomfortably so.

NUTRITION. Give plenty of fluids, such as nourishing broths and juices. Extra vitamins C and A will help fight infection.

For herb teas, homeopathic remedies, and acupressure and massage, see COUGH, BRONCHITIS, and INFECTIONS.

BRONCHITIS

Bronchitis is an inflammation of the larger breathing tubes (bronchi), and usually follows a cold or throat infection. An allergy or stressful situation such as teething or being weaned may lower a child's resistance and lead to bronchitis. There is often a fever of at least 100 degrees F., and the mucus coughed up is usually green or yellow, which means that the infection is bacterial, not viral as in a cold. Bronchitis is usually not severe except in infants or very weak children. The fever usually leaves within four or five days. Although the cough may go on for weeks, it does not usually get much worse than it was at first; if it does, there may be complications that need a doctor's attention.

WHAT A PHYSICIAN MAY DO

A doctor will listen to the chest, lungs, and heart, and examine the ears, nose, and throat. If the cough is very painful or breathing is difficult, he may prescribe cough suppressants or drugs that diminish mucous secretions, hoping to relieve the symptoms. There is no drug really effective against bronchitis. Since it is a self-limited disease, therapy is rarely called for other than rest, use of a vaporizer, natural comfort measures, and good nourishment (mostly in the form of fluids).

WHAT YOU CAN DO AT HOME

PRACTICAL MEASURES. Rest is the most helpful therapy, in a cozy place protected from drafts. Breathing steam from a vaporizer or pot of hot water with juniper or eucalyptus oil, mint, young spruce needles, or catnip in it may bring some relief.

NUTRITION. Give the child lots of broths and juices to drink. Milk (unless it is breast milk) and dairy products should be stopped. Onions, apricots, oranges, radishes, celery, and barley are thought to be especially good for bronchitis.

A good multivitamin and mineral supplement, extra vitamins C, E, A, zinc, calcium, and magnesium will help fight infection.

HERB TEAS. Echinacea, licorice, anise, fennel seed, nettle, raspberry leaf, slippery elm.

For homeopathic remedies and acupressure and massage, see sections on FEVER, COLDS, INFECTIONS, and COUGH.

BRUISES

Children live active lives and often attempt acrobatics and other physical feats they have not yet mastered; because of this, they are continually incurring bruises. Bruises are created when small blood vessels under the skin get crushed by impact and blood escapes into the tissues, causing discoloration. The color changes from red to blue or black to green-yellow or brown, taking up to two weeks to return to normal.

Small children with softer skin show more bruises than older children, and fair-skinned children show bruises more readily than darker ones. Very easy bruising is often a sign of nutritional deficiency, especially of vitamins C or K. Aspirin and other salicylate-containing medications can prevent vitamin K from helping the blood to clot and thus may contribute to easy bruising. Antibiotics can kill the normal benign bacteria in the intestines that create the body's necessary vitamin K. Antibiotics also raise the body's requirements for vitamin C, because of their toxicity.

Unexplained or alarming bruises should be brought to the attention of a physician. Large bruises on the abdomen may imply that an organ has been damaged. Bad bruising on the head may be connected with skull fracture. Bruises whose degree or nature does not fit the child's explanation may be signs of child abuse; the possibility must be explored. If a child seems to fall or bump himself often, problems with his eyes, nervous system, or balance mechanisms may be suspected. Bruises that happen without a fall or physical trauma suggest a clotting disorder. If a child bruises easily, bleeds from the gums and membranes of the nose, has pain in the joints, fatigue, sore throat, anemic symptoms, and a rapid pulse, it is wise to check with a doctor right away; these can be signs of leukemia.

If there has been bad bruising of the face, abdomen, head, or spine, it is a good idea to have a doctor examine the child to check for internal injury.

WHAT A PHYSICIAN MAY DO
The doctor will examine the individual bruises and may also do a full physical exam if she feels this is needed. Eyes and ears may be examined, and simple neurological tests performed to check nerve function and balance. Blood tests may be done to check the

levels of red and white blood cells for indications of anemia, infectious disease, or clotting disorders. The child's general state of health and diet may be discussed, to check for signs of deficiency. The doctor may ask questions about the child's emotional life, parents and other relatives, teachers, friends, and associates if she suspects that the child is being abused.

WHAT YOU CAN DO AT HOME

PRACTICAL MEASURES. With any new injury, it is important to determine how serious the damage is. (See SPRAINS AND STRAINS, FRACTURES, BLEEDING, HEAD INJURIES.) If it seems to be merely a bruise, the first step in treatment is to run cold water over the injured part, or apply a cold wet cloth or a damp cloth with ice inside it, to slow the leakage of blood and decrease the pain and swelling. Keeping cold on the bruise for half an hour would be ideal, but a child is rarely willing to stay still that long. Do not put heat or warm applications on a bruise.

NATURAL APPLICATIONS. If the skin is not broken, an Arnica tincture (diluted 5:1 with water) or an herbal Arnica ointment can be helpful in reducing the depth and discomfort of a bruise. (Herbal Arnica should never be applied to broken skin, as it may cause a rash.)

Poultices of comfrey root, brought to a boil and simmered for five minutes, then cooled and folded in a thin clean cloth, are good for bruises; soothing leaves of mint or wintergreen may be added. Or, a banana skin may be bound over the bruise with the inner side against the child's skin.

NUTRITION. A child deficient in vitamin K, vitamin C, bioflavonoids, zinc, or silicon may bruise easily. Green leafy vegetables, alfalfa sprouts, egg yolk, cultured milk products, and oats are good sources of vitamin K. Foods high in vitamin C and bioflavonoids include citrus fruits, cantaloupe, berries, papaya, pineapple, green peppers, parsley, cauliflower, and broccoli. Zinc-rich foods include seafoods, meats, milk, eggs, nuts, peas, and beans. Silicon is found in oats and most unrefined natural foods. Problems with digestion and assimilation may contribute to deficiencies; check for food allergies. If a child has had antibiotics recently, she should take acidophilus capsules or eat acidophilus-cultured yogurt or kefir for several weeks to restore the balance of healthy flora in the intestines.

Homeopathic Remedies.

Arnica montana (in potentized form, as distinguished from the herb or tincture). The most useful remedy taken internally for bruises. Taken immediately after a fall, it often prevents bruising and soreness.

Pulsatilla. If bruises remain after taking *Arnica* and are primarily in the muscles.

Bryonia. Bruising is primarily in the joints, and the slightest motion is painful.

Rhus toxicodendron. Bruising is mostly in the joints, which are stiff and feel better from motion.

Burns

Burns are tissue injuries caused by heat, chemicals, or electricity. Most burns are first-degree, meaning that the damage is limited to a simple reddening of the skin surface. Second-degree burns show blistering and reach deeper layers of skin. Third-degree burns damage all layers of skin, and often other tissues as well; sometimes the flesh appears charred. In a third-degree burn, nerve endings may be destroyed to the extent that pain will not be felt, and the person may not pull away from the source of the burn. It is vital that the agent causing such a burn be taken away from the skin and the child treated at once for injury and shock; if not, the child's life may be threatened, and the damage irreparable.

Shock often occurs with burns, even those that are not terribly serious. Any time a child gets a burn, have her lie down and rest for a few minutes. If signs of shock are apparent, treat for shock first, then treat the burn itself.

Electrical burns may appear to be small on the surface but are often extensive and severe underneath. If the child has been burned by swallowing or inhaling a chemical or very hot water or steam, it is hard to judge how much damage has been done. If she is in a great deal of pain, or behaves abnormally or goes into shock, a doctor should be consulted immediately.

A child's skin is much more sensitive to heat than an adult's; this means that children can be burned much more seriously, and at lower temperatures. If any burn is very painful for more than two days, it is wise to get a doctor's opinion.

WHAT A PHYSICIAN MAY DO

The doctor will examine the child to find out how much damage has been incurred, to determine the degree of the burns, and to assess complications. Antibiotics, or antibacterial ointments and dressings that must be frequently changed, are often prescribed. At times these may be necessary (as when a bad infection is already established), but doctors sometimes use such treatments preventively. This is not always a prudent practice, since antibiotic treatment can trigger allergic reaction and lower resistance. Infections can usually be prevented by keeping the burned tissues clean and protected. The child's general health should be bolstered through good nutrition and adequate rest.

If burns are serious or extensive, the doctor may decide that hospital care is indicated to facilitate fluid-replacement therapy, pain control through medication, monitoring of infection, and skin grafts. Doctors' opinions vary widely about the proper protocol for treating serious burns. According to author and pediatrician Dr. Lendon Smith, when a child is admitted to the hospital the parents have a right to insist upon certain therapies. For instance, parents may demand that nutritional supplements be given along with the standard intravenous solutions. Dr. Smith recommends that a badly burned child receive 1,000 mg of vitamin C per hour for the first few days, and, daily, 200–500 mg of B-complex vitamins, 100,000 international units of vitamin A, and 90 mg of elemental zinc. These nutrients promote skin healing and help prevent scarring. They are not likely to have toxic effects as long as the amounts are reduced to normal daily doses once healing is well established. Because practices in burn treatment may differ from hospital to hospital, it is important that parents be informed and press for explanations to make sure that their children receive the safest and most effective therapies.

WHAT YOU CAN DO AT HOME

PRACTICAL MEASURES. Treat the child for shock, if necessary (see Shock in Part Two). Immediately remove the agent causing the burn: if the child's clothes are soaked with scalding water, get them off her skin; flush chemicals away with water; if the burn is from the sun, cover her skin with a sheet or light clothing, and move her into the shade or indoors.

Immerse the burned part in ice water, apply an ice pack,

or use the coldest water you can get. Cold will help close the damaged blood vessels below the skin surface and prevent further swelling and fluid loss. Sometimes a first-degree burn can be prevented from becoming second-degree, or a second-degree burn from becoming third-degree, by doing this quickly. Keep the injured body part cold for at least five minutes. If you can, continue until the worst of the pain is gone, or up to an hour. The skin may be damaged by frostbite if ice is left on too long, but if pain returns after the skin has warmed a bit, ice may be reapplied.

Do not let the child become dehydrated. Make sure she keeps drinking plenty of fluids (unless she shows signs of shock; in that case, get help).

If the burn is very bad or covers a large area of the body, the child should receive medical help as soon as possible. Wrap her lightly in a clean sheet or clothing, and use cold applications, if possible, en route to the hospital. If there are any blisters, do not break them. If they are already broken, do not remove the skin. Cover them with a light clean cloth to keep out dirt and reduce the chances of infection.

NATURAL APPLICATIONS. It is generally agreed that burns heal best when kept clean, with air allowed to reach them. Therefore, contrary to many suggested home remedies, it is better not to apply any form of oil or grease to burns. One exception to this is vitamin E oil, squeezed directly from the capsule onto the burned skin; this has been shown to reduce pain, damage, and scarring and to accelerate the healing of many sorts of burns. Note, however, that some brands of vitamin E can sting when applied to burned skin, so it's best to try the oil on a tiny area (or your own burn) first.

Aloe vera gel or juice put directly on the burn is good for pain relief and healing. Comfrey poultices (of leaf, root, or both) applied inside a cool, wet cloth (not directly to the skin, as this may cause a rash) can soothe a burn. Hypericum or calendula tincture (diluted 20:1 with water) may be dabbed on the skin or added to cold soaks.

NUTRITION. Extra vitamins C and E, and calcium lactate, taken internally, can help reduce pain. Vitamin A, B-complex, and zinc are good for healing damaged tissues.

HOMEOPATHIC REMEDIES. *Arnica* should be given first, to reduce the chance of shock. Then, one of the following remedies may be taken every five minutes to an hour, until the pain is reduced or relieved.

Cantharis. Extreme burning pain; child may be anxious, restless, crying, angry.

Causticum. If *Cantharis* does not relieve the pain; child may seem more sad than restless; also a good remedy for pain from old burns.

Phosphorus. Electrical burns.

Urtica urens. Pain, stinging, and itching of burns.

CANCER

A home care book, obviously, is not the place to look for cancer treatments—but prevention of cancer is definitely a part of home care. The rate of cancer among children has been rising drastically, and it is suspected that pollutants and chemicals in the environment, radiation (including X rays and microwaves), medical drugs (given to the mother during pregnancy, or to either parent before conception, as well as to the child), immunizations, and emotional stress may all be contributing to the increase.

Cancer is not one specific disease but a general term that refers to a process of abnormal, rapid, disorderly cell division in some body tissue. The theory is that this occurs when the genetic material of cells (DNA) is traumatized or altered by exposure to chemicals, radiation, or viral influence, and aberrantly sets off the genes responsible for cell growth and division. New growths of tissue (tumors) may be benign, remaining confined to their area of origin and having no serious effects; or malignant, invading other tissues as they grow. Cells may break off and metastasize (travel through the bloodstream to other parts of the body), spreading the cancer.

Warning signs of cancer include: unexplained fatigue, deep bone pain or deep pain anywhere, persistent swollen lymph nodes, muscle weakness, loss of coordination, double vision, unexplained vomiting, unusual bleeding or discharge, extreme changes in bladder or bowel habits, a sore that does not heal, an obvious change in a wart or mole, unusual hardness, lumps, or thickening in any part of the body, difficulty swallowing, and persistent unexplained cough.

It is the opinion of many scientists that cancer cells exist in every human body, but that a healthy immune system consistently is able to overcome them and throw them off. Assuming that this is true, it is important to keep a child's body as strong and pure as possible so his natural resistance is at its best.

Natural approaches to cancer treatment often include a purifying diet: raw foods, fresh fruit or vegetable juices, vitamin and mineral supplementation, and herbs used internally and externally. Unusual nutritive substances, substances isolated from body fluids, and extremes in temperature are sometimes used as anti-cancer agents. Natural therapies seem to have worked against cancer in many cases, but no therapy should be undertaken without expert guidance. Cancer can be extremely serious, and no firm expectations should be held regarding any sort of therapy. The orthodox allopathic approaches such as surgery, radiation, and chemotherapy also seem to work in some cases and fail in others. It is up to the patient and his or her family to decide which route to take. If the standard medical course of treatment is chosen, good nutritional support and healthy life habits should still be observed; these may help the patient resist the unpleasant side effects of treatment and, because they strengthen the child's resistance, may be life-saving.

WHAT A PHYSICIAN MAY DO

Medical treatment will depend upon the type of cancer and the doctor's orientation. The National Cancer Information Service Office can provide the most recent information about standard cancer therapies; the phone number is (800) 4CANCER; (in Alaska (800) 683-6070; in Hawaii (800) 524-1234 on Oahu; call collect from other islands). A number of hospitals and clinics provide nutritional and natural approaches for fighting cancer; some provide these along with orthodox medical treatments such as chemotherapy and radiation. Others provide counseling and survival techniques. More detailed information on alternative therapy can be obtained from the book *Third Opinion: An International Directory to Alternative Therapy Centers for the Treatment and Prevention of Cancer,* by John M. Fink, Avery Publishing Group, 350 Thorens Avenue, Garden City Park, N.Y. 11040.

WHAT YOU CAN DO AT HOME

PRACTICAL MEASURES. Nutrition, rest, exercise, a relaxed and happy environment, and protection from toxic exposure and invasive agents will help keep your child strong. Bottled-up unhappiness and undue ego stress seem to be factors that contribute to low immune function, and to cancer, in human beings of any age. Life can't always go easily, but helping a child talk about his fears or problems, and reassuring him that he is free to have his feelings, can be a tremendous benefit to his health.

To help prevent cancer and to strengthen and detoxify a child's system:

- Avoid *all* unnecessary X rays.
- Avoid *all* unnecessary medications. Most drugs are toxic to some degree and may place extra stress on a child's liver, kidneys, and immune system. Medications thought to be related to a susceptibility to cancer include synthetic hormones, especially estrogens; anabolic steroids; phenacetin (used in some pain killers); methoxypsoralens (used in treatment of psoriasis); and many drugs that are used in cancer therapy. Some drugs do help to save lives and spare people misery at times, but drugs are too often used without enough attention being paid to long-term consequences. Many medications thought in the past to be safe have been withdrawn from use as evidence of their dangers became more apparent. This evidence has too often come in the form of cancer developing in children and adults who trustingly took the drugs prescribed for them.
- Prevent exposure to chemicals, fumes, and pollutants. Keep children away from industrial areas, waste disposal sites, solvents and fluids; do not burn trash containing synthetic materials and plastic.
- Do not smoke in the house, especially near children; do not let children smoke or drink alcohol.
- Protect children against excessive exposure to the sun. Use natural sunscreen lotions and have the child play outdoors at times when the sun is less intense.

NUTRITION. Reduce meat consumption. Some of the by-products of meat digestion are known carcinogens. Commercial meat and poultry are frequently adulterated with hormones and chemicals, and the animals have usually had a very confined and unnatural lifestyle. Use nonmeat sources of protein such as grains, seeds, nuts, legumes, tofu, goat's milk, or fertile eggs. If you do buy meat, make sure it was raised healthfully and organically.

Make sure all foods and juices consumed by the child are free of additives and are as fresh as possible. Try to obtain grains, fruits, and vegetables grown without chemical fertilizers and sprays, these are often labeled as "certified organically grown." Do not use processed foods. Discard any moldy foods or grains.

Raw foods such as fruits, vegetables, greens, nuts, seeds, and sprouted grains should make up as much of the diet as possible. Often recommended as specifically helpful for cancer patients: figs, grapes, red beets, black cherries, carrots, red cabbage, garlic, almonds, asparagus, sesame seeds.

Supplements are usually recommended for support during cancer treatment. A natural balanced vitamin-mineral supplement should be given, along with extra vitamins C, E, B-complex, pantothenic acid, choline, zinc, selenium, vitamin A, and beta carotene. Certain vitamins and minerals (usual and unusual) may be used therapeutically in very large amounts in the treatment of cancer. Expert guidance is important to ensure that there are no untoward side effects.

HOMEOPATHY. A highly experienced homeopath may be able to prescribe a constitutional remedy to strengthen the child's vital force and resistance during cancer therapy.

ACUPRESSURE AND MASSAGE. Rubbing or applying pressure to these points (on both sides) for a minute or so several times a day may help reduce pain and stimulate the immune system. They are not substitutes for therapy but may be used along with other treatment for cancer.

ST 36: A tender point next to the outer side of the big bump at the top of the shin.

SP 6: A tender point three of the child's finger-breadths above the inner anklebone.

KI 1: A point on the sole between the pads of the ball of the foot.
LI 20: The tender points where the creases of the cheek meet the nose
BL 60: A tender point in the hollow behind the outer anklebone, in front of the Achilles tendon.
LV 3: A tender point midway between the first and second metatarsal bones.
LI 4: The point at the end of the crease between the thumb and index finger.

The measures suggested in the above section are intended as natural supports for the child's resistance to disease, **not as cancer therapies.** If a child has had cancer diagnosed, or if it is even suspected, **take prompt but thorough action.** Check with many different kinds of health care professionals, talk to other people who have been through or are going through a similar experience, investigate the possibilities as thoroughly (but as quickly) as possible—then choose the approach that seems best suited to you and your child.

An international support group for parents of children who have cancer that has a chapter in every state of the United States is the Candlelighter's Foundation, 2025 "I" St. NW, Washington, D.C. 20006, (202) 659-5136.

CHICKEN POX

Chicken pox is a common childhood disease, trivial for some children, intensely uncomfortable for others. In general, the younger the child, the less severe the illness. For this reason, many parents make an effort to have their children exposed to chicken pox at the age of two or three.

The illness shows up two to three weeks after exposure. Symptoms are usually fatigue and low fever, like the beginning of a cold. A child may have unexplained diarrhea soon after contact with an infected person; although this is an early warning sign, it is usually not remembered or connected with the chicken pox.

The rash occurs in crops over two to six days. Each crop goes through stages: first, flat red splotches that transform into pimples; next, blisters that are easily broken, forming crusts that itch. Bacterial infection may develop in some of the sores, especially if they are not kept clean or the child scratches a great deal. Badly infected sores may lead to scarring.

Usually the rash is first seen on the scalp or in the mouth, but it soon spreads all over—although some children may have only a blister or two during the whole course of the disease. The fever and contagion usually subside after all the sores are crusted over. A person who has had chicken pox usually retains lifelong immunity to it, although shingles (thought to be caused by the same virus) may sometimes appear in later life.

Complications from chicken pox, such as encephalitis, pneumonia, and Reye's syndrome (a very serious disorder that sometimes follows viral diseases, involving the brain and internal organs) can occur but are rare. Because of the association of chicken pox and aspirin with Reye's syndrome, however, it is best not to give aspirin at all, but to deal with the fever and discomfort in other ways. (See FEVER.)

If your child has mild symptoms and chicken pox is "going around," there is little need to consult a physician. If you are not sure your child has the illness, call your doctor and describe the symptoms. Since chicken pox is highly contagious, it is best not to go to the doctor's office and expose the people in the waiting room. Chicken pox can be very dangerous to infants, persons with low immunity, persons with cancer, and those taking steroid drugs. Of course, if your child's symptoms are alarming (such as vomiting, rapid and shallow breathing, severe headache, extreme stiff neck, convulsions, or unexplained bruised spots or bleeding under the skin), a doctor should be consulted immediately. (See MENINGITIS.)

WHAT A PHYSICIAN MAY DO

A doctor may prescribe acetaminophen (the most common brand name is Tylenol) to bring down fever and ease discomfort of chicken pox. This is preferable to aspirin, which increases the risk of Reye's syndrome, but is nonetheless a questionable practice. And parents should also remember that any use of a drug when not truly needed may do some harm to a growing child's body. Doctors often routinely tell parents to use acetaminophen to reduce their children's fevers, yet it is well known that a moderate fever is the body's natural form of defense against disease. (See FEVER.)

A doctor may also prescribe an antihistamine such as Benadryl to relieve the itching, or topical medications such as calamine lotion or Caladryl (calamine mixed with antihistamine). Antihistamine drugs can have distressing side effects (stupor and disorientation, stomach upset, heart palpitations, agitation, dry mouth, dizziness), and children may develop skin sensitivities to the medication that are worse than the original itching. Because of this, many doctors and parents prefer to control the symptoms by more natural means.

A chicken pox vaccine has recently been developed, made of the live weakened virus *Varicella zoster* that is thought to cause both chicken pox and shingles. Doctors may recommend this for family members who have not had chicken pox. It is unclear at this time how long the immunity will last, whether it will wear off (allowing those immunized as children to later catch the illness at an age when it can be more serious); or whether the "silent" virus in the body will lead to the painful condition of shingles in later life. Parents should be hesitant to risk a vaccine reaction in hopes of preventing an illness as typically mild as chicken pox.

WHAT YOU CAN DO AT HOME

PRACTICAL MEASURES. Make sure the child stays rested and amused; distract her from scratching. If the child can't stop scratching, make sure her fingernails are clean and short and that her hands are washed several times a day. Gloves may help the child to keep from scratching and infecting the sores.

NATURAL APPLICATIONS. To keep the itch under control, soda baths (one-half cup baking soda added to a tub of warm water) may give relief. Some children like cool wet cloths applied to the sores. Adding a warm broth made from boiled oats and barley (one-half cup of each, brought to a boil for twenty minutes in two quarts of water) to bathwater can soothe the sores and speed their drying out.

Sprinkling a mixture of slippery-elm and comfrey root powders on the sores before the scabs have formed can lessen itching. Pastes of baking soda or cornstarch may be dabbed on eruptions.

If there are sores in the mouth, don't give the child sour or salty foods or citrus fruits, which may sting. Soft food is usually best. A rinse or gargle may be made by dissolving one-half teaspoon of salt in one cup of warm water.

Extra vitamin C can provide an antihistamine effect without the adverse results of drugs, and extra vitamins C, A, and zinc help fight infection.

HOMEOPATHIC REMEDIES. In addition to those below, other remedies may be prescribed according to your child's specific symptoms if you consult a homeopathic physician or practitioner.

Antimonium tartaricum. Eruptions are very large and slow to come out; sweating, nausea, or chest congestion; child may be whiny.

Antimonium crudum. Child is irritable and doesn't want to be touched or looked at; touching the spots causes shooting pains.

Apis mellifica. Terrible itching; the skin is pink and puffy; eyelids are swollen; the child feels worse from warmth and is not thirsty.

Belladonna. Headache, fever, hot skin; child finds it hard to sleep.

Pulsatilla. Child is weepy, wants comfort; feels worse in a stuffy room; usually not thirsty even with fever; feels better in open air.

Rhus toxicodendron. Child is restless both mentally and physically, and itching is extreme; muscles may feel stiff and better from motion; eyes may be sticky.

Sulphur. Skin itches, burns and is dry; it is hard for the child not to scratch; feels worse from washing; child may have red lips and irritated anus.

For herb teas and acupressure points, see FEVER and INFECTIONS.

COLD SORES

Cold sores or fever blisters are associated with the herpes simplex virus. Canker sores—nonherpetic ulcers that form on the more movable areas of the mouth lining due to irritation or low resistance—are different, but both may be present at the same time. Cold sores are usually not serious, but in some cases the virus can enter the bloodstream and cause extreme illness that may lead to blindness, nerve damage, even death. This is more likely to happen in infants or people whose immune function is very low. A person with active cold sores should not kiss or share cups or spoons with babies and small children. Anyone who has *ever* had cold sores may be still a carrier, even when there is no active outbreak, and should always exercise caution.

Cold sores usually start with a tingling or itching sensation and reddening of the skin, followed by a blister or group of blisters most often appearing on the lips and around the nostrils (although the first occurrence may be inside the mouth). The blisters develop into whitish, red-edged ulcers that crust over and usually heal within a week or so. Once a person has the herpes simplex virus in his system, stressful situations such as a cold or flu, emotional pressures, intense sun, or fatigue can cause the sores to erupt. Fever often accompanies an outbreak, and sometimes the mouth hurts so much that it is hard to eat and drink.

If fever is very high, or if the outbreak lasts longer than two weeks, a doctor should be consulted.

WHAT A PHYSICIAN MAY DO

The doctor will try to ascertain that the eruptions are of viral origin rather than a bacterial or fungal condition such as trench mouth or thrush. Some doctors more oriented toward natural therapies may recommend supplementing the diet with the amino acid lysine. It is better to have expert guidance if such an approach is chosen; maintaining a correct balance of amino acids in the body is important, especially in growing children.

There seem to be no effective antiviral drugs, so there is not much a doctor can prescribe, except home remedies such as calamine lotion or alcohol, zinc oxide ointment, camphor preparations, or lip balms. Antibiotic ointment may be prescribed to prevent bacterial infection in the sores. Sometimes oral anesthetics are given, but since these deaden feeling in the mouth, they may interfere with swallowing and may cause choking. Many natural health experts think that suppressing skin eruptions with medications is detrimental to overall health. Parents should question the need for any sort of strong prescribed medication.

WHAT YOU CAN DO AT HOME

PRACTICAL MEASURES. Viral infections may be accompanied by fever and malaise. If these are present, the child should be made comfortable, kept warm, and adequately nourished. A vitamin C tablet or acidophilus (in liquid, tablet, or opened capsule form) held directly on the sore or tingling spot may stave off an eruption or make it milder. Applying an ice cube or a hot compress before the blisters begin may do the same.

NUTRITION. Give the child lots to drink. If his mouth is very sore, try ice cubes made of mild juices (cranberry, apple), herb teas (peppermint, lemon balm), or combinations of teas and juices. Avoid citrus fruits, vinegar, and spicy foods, which irritate the sores; also avoid meat, poultry, nuts, and chocolate. A daily multivitamin and mineral supplement is a good idea during any viral infection; extra vitamin C, zinc, and acidophilus can also help.

HOMEOPATHIC REMEDIES.

Arsenicum album. Sores burn intensely; warm liquids relieve the pain; child feels restless but exhausted.

Dulcamara. Sores often appear in cold, wet weather and accompany a cold, sore throat, swollen lymph nodes.

Hepar sulphuris calcareum. Sores very painful; pus may form; child is sensitive to drafts.

Mercurius vivus. Sores and gums may bleed; child has coated tongue, bad breath, swollen lymph nodes, drools in sleep.

Natrum muriaticum. White, pearly blisters on lips, gums, tongue; bothered by anything cold or hot. If given at the early, tingling stage, this remedy may prevent an outbreak.

Rhus toxicodendron. Red blisters around mouth and chin; may be relieved by warm applications; child irritable, sick, achy; feels better from moving around.

ACUPRESSURE AND MASSAGE. (See also FEVER and INFECTIONS.) Rub with the thumb (or press with the thumbnail) the crease where the middle finger meets the palm. Do both hands, several times a day.

COLDS

Most children get several colds a year; symptoms may include runny nose, watery eyes, sore or scratchy throat, moderate fever, sneezing, and coughing. Colds are viral infections that usually occur when the body's resistance to disease is lowered due to fatigue, cold or wet weather, inadequate nutrition, exposure to pollutants and chemicals, or emotional difficulties.

Colds usually last about a week and are thought by some to have a cleansing effect on the system. Occasionally, however, they may lead to complications such as ear infection, sinus infection, bronchitis, or pneumonia. Signs of possible secondary infections include a persistent or deep cough, rising fever, and pain in the ears or chest. Suspect a complication if symptoms get worse rather than better as the days go by. If the child's breathing becomes very rapid (more than forty breaths per minute), or if there is painful coughing, thick yellow-green discharge, diarrhea, abdominal pain, vomiting, rash, or discharge from the eyes that lasts for more than a day or two, telephone a physician.

If a child catches colds frequently or seems almost always to be sniffling and snorting, it is possible that allergy is the culprit. (See ALLERGIES.) Children with weakened immune systems may have frequent colds as well as other illnesses. Fever and coldlike symptoms may also be part of a child's reaction to a DPT, MMR, or other shot. Such reactions should be carefully monitored. Parents are often told that almost any degree of fever and malaise are normal after immunization, leading them to ignore (or be embarrassed to mention) potentially serious conditions.

Remember that a cough or runny nose can be caused by things other than colds—sometimes children put small objects in their noses or get things stuck in their throats or air passages. This can be an emergency; check the throat immediately if a very small child suddenly starts to cough. (See FOREIGN OBJECTS.)

WHAT A PHYSICIAN MAY DO

A doctor will examine the child's ears and throat, listen to her chest, and take her temperature. If complications such as ear infection, tonsillitis, or pneumonia are discovered, treatment will be prescribed (see applicable sections).

Most good pediatricians prescribe warmth, fluids, and rest for colds—things you can prescribe yourself. Some suggest extra vitamins.

Some doctors recommend aspirin to ease discomfort and lower fever, and aspirin is an ingredient of many over-the-counter cold medicines. Parents should be aware that aspirin is not so harmless a substance as many people think: it can cause internal bleeding, and may bring on severe allergic reactions. It is strongly suspected of being connected with Reye's syndrome, a rare but often fatal condition.

Because of aspirin's link with Reye's syndrome, many doctors tell parents to give their children acetaminophen (such as Tylenol) to reduce fever. This is not really a safe medication for children either. Acetaminophen can be toxic; it can damage the liver, and children have been known to die from overdoses. Parents should realize that the fever present in a cold or other ordinary illness is almost always best left alone. The function of fever in the body is to summon the immune elements that fight infection. If a child's temperature is not dangerously high, it is foolish to thwart the body's built-in defenses against disease.

Doctors consulted for colds often prescribe nose drops and decongestants, most of which temporarily alter the condition of the mucous membranes to diminish the amount of mucus produced. These medicines do not hasten the body's recovery. They may actually slow it by suppressing the cleansing process. They do sometimes lessen the symptoms, which may help an exhausted child get some sleep. There are so many cold-related medicines on the market (many of which contain aspirin or alcohol) that it is practically impossible for doctors to have personal knowledge and experience with all of them. Parents should exercise caution about using any medication on their children, no matter how harmless the doctor or drug company literature may say it is; some drugs are dangerous, others may be useless as well.

Some doctors prescribe antibiotics for children with colds, even though antibiotics do not affect viral infections. The rationale behind this is that the antibiotics prevent complications. Parents should be aware that giving a child a toxic drug is not necessarily "preventing complications"; it may be asking for them. Antibiotics have side effects and are toxic to people as well as to bacteria; they should only be used in truly serious situations.

WHAT YOU CAN DO AT HOME

PRACTICAL MEASURES. Make sure the child gets plenty of rest. Provide him with various quiet forms of amusement, and keep him company or read a story from time to time. Don't let him feel alone, but keep other children from getting too close; a cold is usually spread by droplets from coughing or sneezing, or sharing utensils and food.

Keep fresh air circulating. An open window is fine if the child likes it, but don't let the room get chilly. Cool-mist humidifiers or vaporizers may be helpful.

To clear a stuffy head, an herbal steam tent can be devised. Boil a quart or two of water in a pot, then add pinches of aromatic herbs such as wintergreen, mint, rosemary, lavendar, and pennyroyal (or several drops of their oils) and simmer for a minute or two. Pour the liquid into a cool bowl and place it on a steady table or counter so the child can sit beside it and lean his head over to breathe the fumes. If it does not make him feel too claustrophobic, a towel may be draped over bowl, head, and shoulders to help catch the fumes. The steam may feel a little hot at first; make sure the child knows he can sit up straight and breathe cool air whenever he wants to.

Babies may have trouble nursing or sucking from a bottle during a cold because their noses are plugged. Since a tiny child cannot blow her nose, it may be helpful to gently remove the mucus from her nostrils with a rubber suction bulb (found in most drugstores).

NUTRITION. Fluids in the form of juices, herb teas, or broths should be increased. Often children lose their appetites during colds, partly because of swallowing so much mucus and partly because their sense of smell is deranged and things don't taste very good. Don't force a child to eat solid foods, but if she does want to eat, try to avoid giving her milk products, fried or fatty foods, refined sugars and starches. Concentrate on soups, fruits, and vegetables, and include protein from vegetable sources such as tofu, beans, and grains. Garlic, onions, citrus fruits, pineapple, beets, tomatoes, and carrots are excellent foods during colds.

Extra vitamins C, E, A, beta carotene, B-complex, calcium, and zinc will help. Vitamin C has both an antiviral and an antihistamine effect and may be given every few hours until the child is better. For infants, a vitamin C tablet may be crushed to powder and mixed in a spoon with water or added to juice. Give a small amount at first: if a rash appears, there may be something in the tablet to which the baby is sensitive; if so, try a different brand.

Bee pollen is often useful in fighting a cold; give half a tea-spoonful a day. (If the child has never had bee pollen before, give one granule the first day, two the next, up to half a teaspoonful a day; discontinue if the pollen brings on allergy symptoms.)

HERB TEAS. Mint, elder flower, rose hips, lemon slices squeezed in hot water, ginger, peppermint, lemon grass.

HOMEOPATHIC REMEDIES. (See also BRONCHIOLITIS, BRONCHITIS, COUGH, EAR CONDITIONS, FEVER.)

Aconitum napellus. Symptoms come on suddenly, often after ex-posure to cold wind; nose feels dry and stuffy or runs with hot, thin discharge; tension in chest; choking cough; child may be fright-ened and agitated, feverish, chilly, thirsty.

Allium cepa. Clear nasal discharge that burns nostrils and upper lip, stops in open air and runs indoors; red, stinging, watery eyes, teasing cough, sneezing.

Arsenicum album. Frequent colds, sore throats, chest troubles; hot head and cold extremities; white, thin, burning mucus; stopped-up nose unrelieved by lots of sneezing; worse around and after midnight; child is thirsty but drinks in small sips; may feel exhausted but restless.

Baryta carbonica. Colds come on after the child is chilled; runny nose, swollen upper lip, swollen lymph nodes, enlarged tonsils; child may be very shy or a slow learner.

Belladonna. Feverish, flushed, restless; hot face and cold hands and feet; dry nose, watery discharge, hard cough; there may be high fever, throbbing in head and ears, bright red sore throat.

Bryonia. Dry cough that hurts, watery mucus, swollen nose; dry mouth; child may hate to move or be touched, wants to lie still; may dislike company or talking.

Dulcamara. Stopped-up nose, headache, face pain; colds come on after the child has gotten cold and wet or the weather changes.

Euphrasia. Red, watery, irritated eyes; clear nasal discharge and phlegm that causes coughing; better from eating, lying down.

Ferrum phosphoricum. Slight fever, rosy cicles on the cheeks, sneezing; child may be cheerful but gets very tired as evening approaches; better from gentle motion, worse from night and cold. Often staves off a cold if given when first symptoms appear.

Gelsemium. Child is droopy, lethargic, dizzy; achy muscles; headache; nose feels hot and dry inside, with pressure at root. This remedy is often needed in hot weather.

Hepar sulphuris calcareum. Hoarseness, cough, rattling chest, yellowish mucus, sweating; ear troubles; child is very sensitive to drafts, cool air may cause sneezing.

Mercurius vivus. Swollen lymph nodes, chills, sweating, bad breath, foul-smelling mucus; nose feels raw, tonsils or ears may be inflamed; child drools in sleep.

Nux vomica. Stuffy head at night, runny nose in daytime; rough throat, harsh cough; child may be very chilly, constipated, irritable, oversensitive.

Phosphorus. Colds often go to the chest or larynx; one nostril blocked while other runs; nose bleeds; child is imaginative, with many fears; may have high fever without seeming very ill.

Pulsatilla. Thick, bland yellow or greenish mucus; nose runs in open air; child is sensitive and weepy, not usually thirsty; worse in a stuffy room and at night.

ACUPRESSURE AND MASSAGE.

LI 4: The point at the end of the crease between the thumb and index finger.

ST 36: A tender point next to the outer side of the big bump at the top of the shin.

SP 6: A tender point three of the child's finger-breadths above the inner anklebone.

LI 20: The tender points where the creases of the cheeks meet the nose.

COLIC

Colic is, by definition, acute abdominal pain or pain in the large intestine (colon). Colic in babies, however, is merely presumed to be abdominal pain, since it occurs mostly in infants less than four months old who cannot say where or what the problem is.

The main symptom of colic is excessive crying, occurring at the same time every day, notably in the evening, and often lasting for several hours. Since colic often occurs in high-strung and intelligent personalities, and shows a familial tendency, some people think that colic may be a form of abdominal migraine. Some think it is caused by gas, perhaps due to food allergy (even allergy to food the nursing mother is eating) or poor digestion of certain kinds of formula, and that the intolerable pain occurs in the evening because of the baby's exhaustion. Another theory is that general stress during pregnancy causes a loss of potassium in the mother's bloodstream, and as a result the baby's adrenal glands are unstable, causing the period of upset near the end of the day.

Colic is very difficult for everyone. The baby's distress and pain cause concern, while his screaming drives the whole family crazy. The baby's frustration with the colic and the parents' frustration with the screaming can easily make everyone's tension worse. It is difficult, but important, for all family members to remember that the baby cannot help seeming furious, angry, and out of sorts. The parents *can* help it—at least a little; usually something can be done to comfort the baby, even though it may not shorten the episode of colic. Whatever the cause, the baby seems to grow out of it after three or four months, and the colic disappears.

A doctor should be consulted if the baby has been crying constantly for over three hours (unless this is in accord with his established pattern of colic), if the baby is over four months old, if the cry becomes high-pitched or agonized, or if other symptoms of illness (such as fever, chills, vomiting, strange color or blood in the urine or bowel movements) are present.

WHAT A PHYSICIAN MAY DO

A physical examination will be given to check for illness, infection, or any physical discomfort that might otherwise account for the crying. If the child seems healthy and is gaining weight adequately, the main thing a doctor can give is reassurance. Some physicians prescribe a barbiturate such as phenobarbital, to be given about an hour before the colic episode is expected; however, there is now some evidence that phenobarbital used even for short periods decreases a child's learning ability. Antihistamine drugs with sedative side effects may be prescribed. If antihistamines seem to remove the colic, allergy may be the cause.

Parents should realize that the baby could have an allergic response to the drugs themselves, or could—as small children frequently do—respond to a sedative by being further stimulated. (Such a reaction is sometimes an indication of hyperactivity, which is associated with allergy.) The drugs are prescribed, of course, to relieve the baby and make him stop crying, but it's hard to imagine that conscientious parents would choose to expose their baby to drugs with serious side effects, when they know that the colic will last only a few months.

WHAT YOU CAN DO AT HOME

PRACTICAL MEASURES. Try to find something that calms the baby a little bit, even if she continues crying. Walk with her, rub her back, press on her abdomen, give a pacifier, wrap her up snugly, sing or talk to her. Some babies like to lie on their tummies, some like to lie on their backs with their legs bent; some want firm pressure from your hand or a warm hot water bottle on their abdomens; some like to suck on your finger or a bottle or pacifier. Some don't seem to like anything—but if you stay nearby and comfort them, they'll know you're there, caring. Try to care for the baby in shifts, so that one parent isn't doomed to dealing with a baby screaming its head off for hours every evening. Don't blame yourself for feeling tired or irritable—who wouldn't? Sometimes parents think they'd be better off screaming along with the baby. Remember, colic *will* go away someday, and you'll be able to forget (almost) how hard it was.

Be sure to give the baby plenty of company during the day. It has been observed that babies carried in a front-pack several hours a day cry only half as much at night.

NUTRITION. Balanced B-complex vitamins, powdered and mixed in water, added to a bottle or given in a spoon half an hour before the usual time of colic episodes, can help. Calcium-magnesium powder can be given in a bottle the same way. Check the label for adult dosage and give the baby one-tenth of that dose, twice a day.

It is dangerous to give a small baby potassium supplements. Reducing sodium (from salt) in the diet may help preserve potassium. Boiled milk is very high in sodium and incomplete in nutrients for a baby; it should be replaced by a good formula. Check the labels on commercial formulas to be sure they contain essential nutrients, in the right balance, for a growing baby.

Changing formulas may help colic. There are different kinds based on cow's, goat's, and soy milk. Addition of acidophilus culture to the formula can make a difference.

A nursing mother should have a varied, nourishing diet, cut down on salt, and avoid sugar, strong spices, caffeine, foods that cause flatulence, and any foods she suspects of increasing the baby's discomfort. Some nursing mothers who have diligently drunk milk containing synthetic vitamin D (that is, most kinds of milk bought from grocery stores) have found that their babies' colic is reduced when they change to raw or cultured milks, or cut out milk altogether and obtain calcium from other sources such as egg yolk, soybeans, green leafy vegetables, and broths made from fish or chicken (including the bones).

HERB TEAS. (Tepid, not hot): chamomile, dillseed, mint, fennel seed.

HOMEOPATHIC REMEDIES.
    Colocynthis. Baby looks anxious and doubles up from pain.
    Magnesia phosphorica. Warmth and pressure on the abdomen help; baby may pass gas.
    Chamomilla. Baby screams desperately and can only be quieted by being constantly held and walked around the room.

ACUPRESSURE AND MASSAGE.
    LI 4: The point at the end of the crease between the thumb and index finger.
    LI 11: A point at the thumb-side end of the elbow-crease when the arm is bent.
    ST 36: A tender point next to outer side of the big bump at the top of the shin.
    P 6: A point in the mid-forearm, three of the child's finger-breadths above the palm-side wrist-crease.
    · Apply gentle thumb pressure to points about an inch above and below the navel.

CONSTIPATION

Many children have a bowel movement each day, but going for three or four days without one is all right on occasion. However, if the stools are hard and difficult or painful to pass, the condition can be considered constipation. Hard stools may mean that a child is not drinking enough liquid, doesn't have enough fiber in his diet, or is not getting enough exercise. It may be that there is a rash in the anal area or a little tear in the rectum from pushing out hard or large feces, making the child voluntarily hold bowel movements back to avoid more pain. Sometimes excitement, disruption of routine (during travel, for example), worry, and tension inhibit the ordinary working of the bowels.

If there is a lot of pain when the child is trying to move his bowels, if the stools are black or have blood in them, if there is a tear or boil near the rectum or anus, if the child is nauseous or otherwise seems ill and his skin looks yellowish or gray, or if he has had no bowel movement for more than a week and none of the measures mentioned below have helped within a day or two, check with a physician.

WHAT A PHYSICIAN MAY DO

If the constipation does not accompany another illness, the physician will ask questions about diet, bowel habits, emotional stresses in the child's life, and then examine the abdomen and rectum for blockage, pain, rashes, or tearing. Some may recommend the use of glycerin suppositories or oral laxatives. Some will advise a change in diet.

Sometimes doctors, curious to see their patients' insides, order lower bowel X rays. Parents should remember that, especially for children, such X rays are hardly ever justified—only if severe blockage or tumors are suspected. Unless the constipation is painful and long-standing, no other cause has been found, and nothing else has worked to relieve it, it is best to spare your child the radiation.

WHAT YOU CAN DO AT HOME

PRACTICAL MEASURES AND NUTRITION. Improving the child's diet and fluid intake is usually enough to get rid of constipation. Have him drink a large glass of water an hour before each meal. Don't give him refined or sugary foods; have him eat lots of fresh fruits, vegetables, and whole grains, but temporarily stop rice products. Replace cow's milk with cultured milks such as yogurt and kefir or with goat's milk, or eliminate milk altogether.

A balanced B-complex (including pantothenic acid, inositol, and choline), vitamins A, D, E, K, C, and magnesium work to keep the bowels in order.

For an uncomfortable, or long-lasting case, try mixing a tablespoonful each of olive oil and lemon juice and have the child sip it, followed by cups of hot water and lemon juice throughout the day. Prune juice or black cherry juice (or concentrate) can act as laxatives. Add prunes, figs, tomato juice, bran, flax seeds, and sesame products to the diet.

It is best to avoid mineral oil (which robs the body of oil-soluble vitamins A, D, E, and K), laxatives (which work at first but may make the body depend on them to move the bowels), and enemas (which can damage the lining and muscle fibers of the lower intestine).

Having a regular time to sit on the toilet is helpful to some children. Some children need routine in order to relax; others dislike regimentation.

Remember that children need exercise. A couch potato or avid scholar may need to be urged to go out for a walk or a game of basketball.

HERB TEAS. Comfrey, raspberry leaf, papaya, ginger, licorice root.

HOMEOPATHIC REMEDIES. Use these only if constipation is very troublesome and diet changes do not relieve it.

Bryonia. Large, dry stools that are hard to push out; stitching pains; child is dry-mouthed, thirsty, and grumpy.

Calcarea carbonica. Child may feel better when constipated; large stools, first hard, then sticky, then liquid; child may sweat easily, have clammy hands and feet.

Causticum. Unsuccessful, painful straining to move the bowels; child's face may turn red; stools may be narrow, mucusy, pass better standing up.

Graphites. Balls of feces stuck together with mucus; anus aches after passing stool; child may be overweight and have skin problems.

Lycopodium. Passing stools may be painful; abdomen is bloated, full of gas; child may have ravenous appetite
but become full quickly; warm drinks relieve discomfort.

Natrum muriaticum. Dry, crumbly stool; bleeding anus; child may crave salt, be depressed or emotional, dislike consolation.
Nux vomica. Frequent urge to pass stool, but only a small amount comes out; worse after spicy or stimulating food; child is irritable; better in the evening.
Silicea. Straining without success; the feces may begin to come out, then go back in; child may be easily tired, anxious, or shy.
Sulphur. Child's skin may look dirty, worse from washing; stools hard; anus red, burning; child may be self-centered, curious.

ACUPRESSURE AND MASSAGE.
  · Massage, in a clockwise direction, the area around the navel, extending outward two or three inches in all directions.

CONVULSIONS (Seizures)

Convulsions are episodes of unconsciousness accompanied by uncontrolled muscle contraction. The child's body stiffens, with arms and legs jerking, eyes staring or rolled back in the head; this may be followed by sudden collapse. Most convulsions last only a few minutes. (Of course, even one minute can seem long and terrifying to the person watching.) Convulsions are caused by an altered electrical discharge in the nervous system, a phenomenon that may have many different sources. In children, the trigger is usually a quickly rising fever; the cause may occasionally be poisoning, a breath-holding spell, a head injury, an infection that involves the nervous system (e.g., meningitis or encephalitis), epilepsy, or—very rarely—a tumor or defect in the nervous system.

Approximately one child in twenty has at least one convulsion before the teens; most of these occur between the ages of six months and four years, probably because the nervous system is immature. Even though it is likely that the convulsion is not dangerous and has no serious underlying cause, it is important to protect the child during the episode and to find out why it happened.

Any child who has had a seizure should be checked by a doctor to rule out any serious underlying cause. It is a good idea to telephone a doctor right away, although the examination does not necessarily have to happen immediately (especially if the convulsion accompanies fever). If the child does not quickly regain consciousness, is having trouble breathing, or seems to be very ill, see a doctor immediately.

WHAT A PHYSICIAN MAY DO

The doctor will ask questions about what happened during the convulsion to try to find out whether neurologic defect, illness, or poisoning might have caused it. A physical exam will be given. Especially if the child has been very ill—with fever, stiff neck, and lethargy—a lumbar puncture (spinal tap) may be done to check the spinal fluid for evidence of meningitis or encephalitis. An EEG (brain-wave evaluation) may be performed a week or more after the seizure, to look for nervous system abnormalities. Sometimes a doctor will want a child to stay in the hospital for further evaluation, especially if the child is less than six months old. Try to arrange it so that you can stay with the hospitalized child.

If a seizure has lasted longer than a few minutes and the child has been brought to the emergency room or doctor's office and is still convulsing, an injection of phenobarbital or a related drug may be given to stop it. There is a lot of controversy about giving seizure-controlling drugs regularly to children who have had simple febrile seizures. Once she is taking the drug, it is unlikely that the child will convulse the next time she has a fever—but it's quite possible that she wouldn't have, anyway.

If drug therapy seems to be necessary because of frequent, severe seizures that do not seem to be affected by safer therapies, it is best to find a doctor experienced in dealing with children's seizures. Convulsions can be a scary thing, especially if they are frequent or seem to have no simple explanation. When getting a medical evaluation, however, it is important to remember that some doctors, in their pursuit of information, have no reservations about subjecting children to frightening tests, hospitalization, and separation from parents. Consult several doctors until you find one who is both intelligent and sympathetic.

CONVULSIONS

WHAT YOU CAN DO AT HOME

PRACTICAL MEASURES. Stay with the child and keep her from getting hurt. Turn her onto her side, or on her front with her head turned—preferably on a clear area of the floor (where there is nothing to bump against) rather than a bed, from which she might fall. *Don't* try to control the jerking or to put an object between her jaws to prevent her biting her tongue; this rarely does any good, and might cause an injury. Don't give her a pillow: keeping the head at a low level will help drain saliva or mucus so she doesn't choke. Pull on her jaw gently to extend her neck (chin turned upward from the chest) to keep the airway open so she gets enough oxygen.

Try to keep calm, and watch carefully so you can remember details of the convulsion and report accurately to the doctor. Had the child been holding her breath or hyperventilating before the seizure began? Did it start with several moments of blank staring? Did the skin look gray, or pale, or flushed? Did the muscle contractions involve both sides of the body? Where did they start, and did they move to other parts? Were (or are) there any symptoms such as panting or vomiting that might suggest poisoning? Is there fever? If the cause is fever, you may want to lower it a little bit to comfort the child—and yourself—after the convulsion is over. Remember, however, that fever is not in itself a bad thing. The body produces the high temperature to fight off infection; therefore you should not attempt to reduce it too much. Uncovering the child, and sponging her with cool water or cooled mint tea may lower the fever enough. Never put a child who is having or has just had a convulsion in the bathtub, or give any medicine by mouth.

NUTRITION. The following nutrients may help prevent convulsions. They should be given as part of the child's daily diet, *not* as treatment for a current seizure: vitamin C, balanced B-complex, calcium and magnesium, zinc, and lecithin. Hypoglycemia and allergies may be related to seizures.

HOMEOPATHIC REMEDIES. For remedies related to febrile seizures, see FEVER. Note: A convulsion will usually end before a remedy can be given. Do not put pellets or drops into an unconscious child's mouth, as they may be inhaled. Crush the pellet or dissolve it, then touch the powder or liquid to the lining of the mouth. A child who has convulsions may benefit from a constitutional remedy chosen by an experienced prescriber.

ACUPRESSURE AND MASSAGE. *During a seizure:*
· Pinch the child's earlobe between your thumb and index finger.
  GV 26: Press your thumbnail into the space between the child's nose and lip.
    Cranial manipulations have been of benefit to children with a tendency to seizures. Consult an experienced craniosacral therapist, chiropractor, or osteopath.

COUGH

Coughing is a useful reflex action of the body, designed to clear air passages of foreign substances or excess secretions. Because of this, it is foolish to artificially suppress a cough unless it is extremely violent or painful and keeps a sick child from getting enough air or rest. A cough is usually a response to a tickle or irritation in the throat due to a cold, sore throat, or bronchitis, postnasal drip from an allergy, or teething in the lower jaw. Sometimes it is part of an episode of asthma, or a sign of a more serious respiratory infection such as pneumonia or whooping cough (see appropriate sections).

Indications that a respiratory condition needs medical attention are: difficult, noisy, painful breathing; sucking in of the lower ribs; flaring nostrils; and bluish discoloration of the face, lips, or nailbeds. Fever with rapid respiration (more than forty breaths per minute in a child over one year old, thirty per minute in a child over six, and twenty-five per minute in a child over ten) usually means an infection.

If the sounds that accompany the cough are loose and rattly, from the upper middle of the back or chest, this usually means that there is a lot of extra mucus in the larger, upper breathing tubes, and that the disease is probably not too serious. Quiet, whistling sounds (wheezing) usually mean that swollen tissues or secretions are blocking lower, middle-sized airways; these are heard (especially on breathing out) in asthma and bronchiolitis. If the deepest lung tissues are full of fluids, as in pneumonia, the sounds will be very soft, like tissue paper being crumpled.

If much coughing occurs in very young infants, a doctor should certainly be consulted, since it may mean a serious lung problem.

WHAT A PHYSICIAN MAY DO

To ascertain whether the cough is caused by infection, a foreign object, or some other abnormality, the doctor will give a physical exam with special attention to throat, nose, and ears, and listen to the chest with a stethoscope. If the cause is infection, the doctor may try to determine its severity by means of X rays, sputum cultures, or blood tests.

Since many doctors order chest X rays routinely to check for pneumonia, it is up to the parents to ask pointed questions to be sure the radiation exposure is justified. Do the child's other symptoms indicate serious lung involvement? Would the X ray give information that would make a difference in treatment, or would the child most likely be treated in the same way, X ray or not?

Doctors often prescribe medications such as expectorants, antihistamines, and cough suppressants to control cough and its accompanying symptoms. These drugs are often of little value and can have side effects. Should the cough appear to be caused by bacterial infection, many doctors give antibiotics. Most respiratory ailments are viral, however, and antibiotics are only effective against bacteria.

WHAT YOU CAN DO AT HOME

PRACTICAL MEASURES. If there is no sign of sickness, and the coughing is violent or the child seems to be suffocating or turning pale or blue, check to see if an object has been inhaled or is lodged in the throat. If you find one, reach in and pull or hook it out with your fingers. If this can't be done, hold the child upside down and give a sharp slap between the shoulder blades. If this is not enough, call 911. (See also FOREIGN OBJECTS, and Emergencies in Part Two.)

For coughs accompanying respiratory infections, drinking large amounts of fluid can thin and loosen secretions, as well as help with fever and dehydration.

A cool-mist vaporizer can soothe irritations in the throat and air tubes and help loosen phlegm. If the air in the house is too hot or dry, turn on the shower to let mist billow out and add moisture to the air, or boil water on the stove. Herbs or oils may be added to the water: young spruce needles, eucalyptus, juniper, mint, or catnip.

Soothing the throat with a mixture of honey and lemon juice, given by spoon or mixed with hot water and sipped, may give relief. Drugstore cough medicines are often full of sugar and may contain aspirin or cough-suppressing drugs. The active ingredient in many cough syrups is alcohol, which children should not have. Natural food stores sell sugar-free cough syrups, some of which children can stand.

NUTRITION. Extra vitamins C, A, E, and zinc are helpful during any respiratory infection. Garlic, onions, Jerusalem artichokes, parsley, alfalfa sprouts, black currants, black cherry juice, steamed pears, dried apricots, and soups made with barley are good. Chewing licorice root is soothing if the child likes the taste.

HERB TEAS. Ginger, coltsfoot, dillweed, horehound, elecampane, thyme.

HOMEOPATHIC REMEDIES.

Aconitum napellus. Very sudden onset, often after being in cold wind; child is very anxious; cough may wake child from sleep and is usually sharp, short, dry, croupy.

Antimonium tartaricum. Bubbling or rattling of mucus in chest, child is sweaty, drowsy, or dizzy and may have heart palpitations; better from sitting up, burping.

Belladonna. Teasing cough as if from a tickle or speck in the throat; violent bouts of coughing makes the head feel about to burst; red face, hot skin, dilated pupils.

Bryonia. Cough hard, dry, hurts; child is thirsty, grumpy, doesn't like to move, holds head and chest when coughing; worse in the daytime; better from rest.

Drosera. Spasms of tickling, dry cough lead to retching; yellow expectoration, nosebleed; child holds his sides; worse at evening and night, worse lying down.

Ferrum phosphoricum. Short, tickly, painful cough; child is tired with flushed face. This remedy is good early in any respiratory infection.

Hepar sulphuris calcareum. Cough is loose, rattly, gagging, or comes in long, dry jags, child is sensitive to drafts, bends head backward; better in a warm, moist atmosphere.

Kali bichromium. Brassy, hacking cough that raises sticky, ropy yellow mucus; worse in early morning, from eating, drinking, or open air; better from warmth.

Nux vomica. Dry, teasing cough with soreness in the chest and retching; child is irritable, shivery, oversensitive to noise; worse after eating or drinking.

Phosphorus. Hoarse, tickly larynx; cough is worse from laughing, cold air; tightness in chest; exhaustion; headache; child is better from rubbing, company; wants cold drinks, but may vomit when liquids warm up in the stomach.

Pulsatilla. Cough is dry in the evening and loose in the morning; thick green or yellow mucus; worse in a stuffy room or lying down; child is clinging, weepy.

Rumex crispus. Teasing, hacking cough that prevents sleep; frothy or stringy expectoration; chest sore in middle or left side; worse from cold air and uncovering.

Spongia tosta. Loud, sawing, barky cough; worse from talking; chest feels weak; child awakes feeling suffocated and anxious; worse from warmth, lying down.

ACUPRESSURE AND MASSAGE.

CV 22: A point in the notch at the base of the throat, just above the breastbone.

LU 1: A tender point in the indentation below the shoulder end of collarbone.

· Rub the point in the pad of the palm below the crack between middle and index fingers.

· Rub the point in the pad of the palm below the index finger, next to the base of the thumb.

CROUP

Croup is difficulty in breathing that comes on as a result of inflammation and swelling of the larynx and upper air passages. Associated with viral infection, it is distinguished by raspy breathing and a loud, hard, hacking, ringing, or seal-like barking cough. Some children become croupy every time they have a cold; others have only one or two episodes. It is usually outgrown by adolescence as the child's breathing tubes enlarge.

Croup may develop over a period of days, but it can often wake a child in the middle of the night. He may be quite frightened because it is so hard to breathe. Unless croup is accompanied by high fever (103 degrees F. or more) or severe symptoms of suffocation, it can usually be relieved by home care measures.

If the fever is high, or breathing seems to be dangerously obstructed (signs of this are: sitting forward with the head tilted and jaw pointed outward; gasping or drooling; skin that looks bluish or dusky), the child should be taken to the emergency room right away in case he has *epiglottitis,* a bacterial infection that can completely cut off breathing.

WHAT A PHYSICIAN MAY DO

The doctor will try to determine whether it is epiglottitis rather than simple croup. If it is, the child will be given oxygen, or a tube may be inserted to ensure that she can breathe. Antibiotics will be given intravenously. The child will be kept in a room with high humidity to ease breathing during recovery.

If it is only croup, the child may be put in a room or under a tent with vaporizers. Since it is usually just as easy to humidify the air at home as at the hospital (and much cheaper and much less stressful), as soon as you are sure there is no emergency, take the child home.

WHAT YOU CAN DO AT HOME

PRACTICAL MEASURES. Keep the child calm, as panic and sobbing will make breathing even more difficult. Cool, moist air will often reduce the swelling of the air passages right away. Take the child to an open window and let her breathe fresh air; or have her stand and breathe in front of the open refrigerator, or use a cool-mist vaporizer; turn on the shower or boil water in an open kettle to fill the air with mist. Then sing a song or read a story to comfort her; have her sit on your lap to raise her up a bit, since steam will rise in the air. After the attack subsides, keep the air moist so recurrence is unlikely. If natural measures do not give relief within ten to twenty minutes, call ahead to an emergency room and take the child in. The cool night air pouring through the open car window is often enough to stop the attack; if this happens, turn around, go back home, and call to report it was a false alarm. Don't be embarrassed to call again if you need to. Even if the hospital staff act officious, the hospital's purpose is to help you when you need it.

HOMEOPATHIC REMEDIES. (See also COUGH and FEVER.)
Aconitum napellus. Croup accompanied by extreme fear and agitation; often comes on after being in cold, dry air.
Spongia tosta. Sudden waking in the night, coughing with a sawing sound; made worse by talking.
Hepar sulphuris calcareum. Child is chilly, with a loose, rattly cough; or croup continues after other remedies have helped a little.
Sulphur. Loose cough, rattling mucus, spits up green, pus-like sputum; soles of the feet may burn.

For acupressure and massage, see COUGH and FEVER.

CUTS AND SCRAPES

Most cuts, scrapes, and wounds that children get are not serious and heal quickly—all you have to do is keep them clean. Sometimes, though, a wound can be big or deep, or contain foreign matter that is hard to thoroughly clean out. If a wound occurs on the face, abdomen, chest, or back, or seems to involve deeper tissues than skin (tendons, muscle, nerves, larger blood vessels), it is a good idea to get professional care to ensure healing without infection or bad scarring. Possible emergencies include: any wound that is seriously bleeding (see BLEEDING); any puncture wound; a gaping or jagged cut; a cut on the face or any body part on which it might be difficult to keep the edges neatly closed; any large wound that will not stay closed with tape or adhesive telfa pads and might require stitches. If there is weakness or tingling in a wounded arm or leg, or if for more than twenty-four hours a wound is red, swollen, forming pus, intensely tender, and accompanied by fever, check with a physician.

WHAT A PHYSICIAN MAY DO

If it is a large, deep, or very dirty wound, the doctor will thoroughly clean and examine the area to check for any tendons, muscles, blood vessels, or nerves that might need repair. If minor surgery or stitches are necessary, the doctor may give an anesthetic. If your child has ever shown allergic symptoms when given lidocaine, novocaine, or any of the "-caine" drugs, make sure the doctor does not use any of these. If complicated surgery is necessary (to repair a serious wound on the hand or face, for example), try to find other people who have had such operations to recommend a surgeon. Surgeons' talents vary considerably, and a botched job may mean an ugly scar or permanent impairment.

Some physicians give tetanus shots for every wound that breaks the skin. Only puncture wounds or wounds that have dirt deep inside, closed off from contact with air, can cause tetanus. Unnecessary shots are dangerous. (See Immunizations in Part Two.)

Some doctors prescribe antibiotics or antibiotic ointments for wounds that might become infected. Because there are dangers in using antibiotics, even topically (some research has shown they may even slow wound healing), it is best to wait, keep the wound clean, and use medication only if a bad infection actually develops.

WHAT YOU CAN DO AT HOME

PRACTICAL MEASURES. For a wound that is not an emergency, the first step in treatment should be to hold the injured part under a gentle stream of cold water. This will lessen the pain and panic and will also help cleanse the cut. After a few minutes of this, you may be able to wash the wound with soap and warm water, taking care to get out all grit, dirt, and debris. If it would be uncomfortable to leave the cut uncovered, or it is likely to get dirty, put on clean gauze or a comfortable bandage. If the child needs a Band-Aid for psychological support, give him one, but take it off as soon as possible, so air will harden the scab and help it heal.

Keep wounds clean and dry. Don't use greases or ointments that will keep a protective scab from forming. It's all right to apply mild antiseptic, but avoid iodine and Merthiolate; they sting, and are strong enough to damage the tissues.

Calendula tincture (diluted 5:1 in clean water) is effective against infection (or fresh calendula juice if you can get it).

Lemon juice is also a disinfectant. If the wound is deep and doesn't close, use diluted hypericum tincture. The herbs echinacea and goldenseal can be brewed and used as a wash, or applied in the form of powder.

If redness and swelling develop around a wound, apply a poultice of clean raw grated potato, echinacea (stewed in warm water), or fresh comfrey leaves (wrapped in a thin clean cloth; don't touch the skin as the prickles may cause a rash). Leave poultices on for half an hour, repeating as needed.

For herb teas, homeopathic remedies and acupressure and massage, see INFECTIONS.

DEHYDRATION

Dehydration is the loss of too much water from the body. If a person's tissues lose more water than is replaced, the chemical (electrolyte) balance in the bloodstream can be upset, and shock may be the result. Babies and small children are likely to become dehydrated very quickly because of their small size, relatively large surface area, and high rate of metabolism. High fever, vomiting, and diarrhea can cause dehydration in children; so can excessive sweating (for instance, during hot weather or very strenuous exercise) or a very low intake of liquids.

If a child is losing water in any way, it is vital that the fluids be replaced. Weight loss should never be attempted by causing dehydration—it is extremely dangerous to the child's health, and any weight lost would be from body water, not from fat. Teenagers have died of dehydration due to rigorous sports "training" techniques, such as running laps in rubber suits, or losing weight by going without salt and water. Unfortunately, coaches and teachers do not always understand the risks and may encourage these practices.

Symptoms of dehydration are: infrequent, scanty, dark-colored urine (don't forget that B vitamins can harmlessly make the urine bright yellow); a pinched face with the nose appearing sharp and prominent; easily wrinkled, old-looking skin (to test this, gather some abdominal skin in your fingers and release it; during dehydration, the skin loses its elasticity and does not spring back); dry mouth and lips, sunken eyes, or, in an infant, a sunken fontanel (the "soft spot" on top of the head).

If any of these symptoms are present and are not corrected right away by giving fluids (especially if the child refuses to drink), a doctor should be consulted immediately.

WHAT A PHYSICIAN MAY DO

The lost electrolytes and fluids will be replaced—intravenously, if necessary. Shock and any other extreme conditions (vomiting, diarrhea, fever) will be treated.

WHAT YOU CAN DO AT HOME

PRACTICAL MEASURES. If a child has fever, vomiting, diarrhea, or is sweating a great deal, give him as much liquid (juices, broths, water) as he will take. This will help to prevent dehydration. Keep it up even if he vomits most of what he takes; a little bit of water is being retained, and he is better off having the liquid than not. Sucking on an ice cube or frozen juice bar is sometimes easier.

If a child is clearly dehydrated, give him frequent sips of a drink made in these proportions: 1 quart of water + 2 tablespoons of honey (or sugar) + 1/4 teaspoon salt + 1/4 teaspoon baking soda. Also give small sips of orange juice, or banana blended in orange juice. Drops of liquid chlorophyll may be added. The solution should be quite dilute, since water is the substance a dehydrated person needs most, and should not taste very salty. Salt replaces the sodium and chloride lost by the body; soda gives carbonate; oranges, bananas, and chlorophyll give potassium; fruits, honey, or sugar give calories for fuel. If the dehydrated child is an infant, have him nurse constantly if this is possible; if not, give the solution in a bottle or from a spoon. If the child seems unable to take this fluid or to keep it down, or if he is drinking it but it seems not to be helping, consult a doctor. If shock occurs, call 911 or go immediately to an emergency room. (See Emergencies in Part Two.)

DIABETES

Diabetes mellitus ("sugar diabetes") is a condition in which the pancreas is unable to produce or efficiently use insulin—the hormone that enables the body to use glucose (the breakdown product from sugars and starches). Without enough insulin, glucose cannot be used by the brain and body cells; it builds up in the blood and spills over into the urine. Because of this disruption in metabolism, the fats and proteins in the person's tissues begin to break down excessively in the body's attempt to obtain some fuel. This can cause ketoacidosis, a dangerous condition that may lead to coma or even death.

Complications of uncontrolled diabetes include: low resistance, susceptibility to infections, slow wound-healing and gangrene (due to poor circulation), nerve disorders, muscle wasting, kidney damage, blindness (from cataracts, glaucoma, and damage to the blood vessels of the retina), and heart and artery disease.

Diabetes in children is usually more severe than the type first discovered in adulthood. In children, the symptoms of diabetes may include: frequent need to urinate; extreme thirst; sweet, fruity-smelling breath; nausea, vomiting; shortness of breath; and possibly coma. These may show up unexpectedly, before any sign of the disease is apparent even in a medical exam. Other symptoms may be ravenous hunger, weight loss, blurry vision, cramps, numbness and tingling, itching skin, frequent infections, and sores that heal very slowly.

Symptoms of diabetes may occur because of actual damage to the pancreas through inflammation, scarring, or tumors, but they can also be caused by impaired function of other glands such as the adrenals or thyroid. Symptoms of diabetes are made worse by a high intake of refined carbohydrates (sugar and white flour) and hydrogenated fats (in shortening and processed foods such as cookies, candy, peanut butters, margarines, and cheeses).

Childhood-onset diabetes is potentially such a serious disease that a physician's guidance is indispensable. Administration of insulin or oral diabetic medications will probably be necessary, however, and control of blood sugar can be enhanced through diet and exercise, which improves the body's ability to use glucose.

WHAT A PHYSICIAN MAY DO

Unless the case is first discovered by an emergency event such as ketoacidosis or coma, diagnosis is usually made by means of blood tests (glycohemoglobin, or the glucose tolerance test) and urine tests for sugar. (Urine tests can show a false positive result if the child has recently taken a lot of vitamin C.)

Doctors treat diabetes with a combination of diet, exercise, and medications—usually injections of insulin. Daily use of tablets or dipsticks to test the child's urine for sugar or ketones or test-strips designed to test the blood-glucose level from a drop of blood from the fingertip may be required. Parents will be instructed in correct monitoring of insulin. An overdose may cause an insulin reaction, the symptoms of which are faintness, sweating, irritability, hunger, pallor, or drowsiness; this can be counteracted by giving concentrated glucose, sugar, or fruit juice right away. Careful control of diabetes can help reduce the likelihood of severe complications.

WHAT YOU CAN DO AT HOME

PRACTICAL MEASURES. Diabetes is too serious a problem to be treated with home remedies; expert assessment and advice are needed. However, good nutrition and regular exercise such as swimming, hiking, bike-riding, or dancing can improve a child's body functions and resistance, making the need for medication less drastic. A child should always have something light to eat before exercising, and fruit juice or other sources of carbohydrates should be available during and after exertion.

NUTRITION. The child should eat small, frequent meals that consist of unrefined, unprocessed natural foods, especially whole grains, fresh fruits and vegetables, high-quality protein, nuts, and seeds. Cucumbers, bananas, green beans, Jerusalem artichokes, buckwheat, brewer's yeast, and cold-pressed vegetable oils are helpful to diabetics. B-complex vitamins, including B_{12} and niacin, vitamins C and E, and chromium and potassium are especially needed.

HERB TEAS. Raspberry leaf, chicory, dandelion, fenugreek, nettle.

ACUPRESSURE AND MASSAGE.

   SP 21: A very tender point below the middle of the armpit, at nipple level; rub both sides with several flat fingertips.

   KI 3: The tender point just behind the upper rear aspect of the inner anklebone.

   KI 1: A point on the sole between the pads of the ball of the foot.

   LU 7: The tender point on the undersurface of the thumb-side forearm bone two of the child's thumb-widths above the palm-side wrist-crease.

   · Massage all tender points along the muscle ridge that runs from neck to shoulder.

DIAPER RASH

Anyone who wears diapers is likely to get a rash on the bottom at some time or another, but certain babies' skins are particularly sensitive. Most rashes are due to irritation from contact with urine and stools, but once the skin is irritated, a bacterial or fungal infection may complicate the rash. Sometimes a baby's skin is sensitive to soaps or detergents, or chemicals in lotions, powders, or disposable diapers. A rash may be an allergic reaction to food eaten by the baby or by the nursing mother.

   If diaper rash is seriously infected, develops into boils or blisters, or spreads beyond the diaper area and can't be controlled by natural measures, take the baby to a doctor.

WHAT A PHYSICIAN MAY DO

The doctor will look the baby over to make sure he is generally healthy, and examine the rash. A skin-scraping may be taken to determine whether the problem is bacterial or fungal. For severe cases, some doctors prescribe steroid creams or antibiotics, which may or may not relieve the misery. These drugs can interfere with growth and often have dangerous side effects, so try all other methods diligently.

WHAT YOU CAN DO AT HOME

PRACTICAL MEASURES. Have the baby wear loose diapers or go without them as often as possible so air can circulate. Do not use plastic pants or plastic-coated disposable diapers except in special circumstances (traveling, visiting a royal palace) when an accident with a leaky diaper would be disastrous. Use several diapers instead, especially at night, and woolen diaper-covers (found in baby shops and catalogues); these don't trap the hot, wet urine against the skin to "cook" the way plastic pants can.

Avoid all but the mildest soaps when bathing the baby; soap can wash away the skin's protective oil. Wash diapers in mild laundry soap or detergent. Give the diapers an extra rinse to get out soap residues, adding half a cup of white vinegar to reduce ammonia formation. Don't use lotions, creams, or disposable wipes containing alcohol, fragrances, and other chemicals.

If the baby's urine seems very concentrated (dark or smelly) and therefore more irritating, it can be diluted by giving her more to drink. If certain foods cause diarrhea or seem to make the baby's skin irritated, eliminate them for several months and see if there's any change.

Check for wet or dirty diapers frequently so they can be changed right away. Wash the baby's bottom with warm water, or wipe the skin with clean oil before putting on a dry diaper. Mineral oil, which is often found in commercial baby oils, should not be used; it can leach the oil-soluble vitamins A, D, E, and K from the child's body right through the skin. Cold-pressed, unrefined oils such as olive oil are good substitutes.

NATURAL APPLICATIONS. Most diaper rashes caused by irritation or bacterial infection can be soothed by the application of calendula ointment, or aloe vera gel and goldenseal salve. These can be found in natural food stores or baby shops; if you can't find them, ask a store to order some. Ointments containing zinc oxide, such as Desitin, or petroleum-based ointments like Vaseline are commonly used against diaper rash; these are useful as protection, but delay healing if they are put on skin that is already irritated.

If a rash is fiery red with distinct, raised borders, and appears to spread from the anal area or concentrate in skin folds, it may be a yeast infection. This can be combatted by having the child take acidophilus, which can be given in the form of powder or liquid (also pulverized tablets or contents of capsules) mixed with liquid and given by spoon; it is also found in cultured milks such as yogurt and kefir. B vitamins, especially niacinamide, are helpful. If a baby is nursing, the mother should also supplement her diet with B-complex and acidophilus. Acidophilus mixed in water, or yogurt, may be applied as a poultice to the skin. One home remedy long in use for yeast infection is gentian violet, a nontoxic dye (available in drugstores) with which the spots are painted; this gives the skin and diapers a dramatic purple color, but sometimes stops a troublesome eruption and is safer than drugs. A wash made of bay leaves (three or four simmered in a cup of water for fifteen minutes, then cooled and applied) can help control yeast infection.

Diarrhea

Diarrhea—very loose, very frequent movement of the bowels—is one of the body's methods of cleansing itself of harmful or irritating substances such as germs, toxins, and allergens. The presence of an irritant causes the muscular walls of the intestines to contract more intensely than usual, cutting down absorption of all substances, including fluids and nutrients. It is normal for nursing infants to have six or eight loose stools a day; this is not diarrhea. Real diarrhea is usually watery and has a green tinge from bile that is rushed through the intestines so quickly it doesn't turn brown, as it normally would. It may occur only once in a day or, depending on the cause, go on for days or weeks, in some degree.

The main dangers posed to a child by diarrhea are dehydration and mineral or electrolyte imbalance (see DEHYDRATION). Other signs that the condition may be serious are: diarrhea lasting longer than three or four days without improvement; weight loss; the presence of blood or pus in the stools; other symptoms of illness or poisoning, such as high fever, intense pain, listlessness, or vomiting. If the irritant causing the diarrhea is a poison or infective agent, the cause must be recognized and dealt with.

Common causes of diarrhea in infants and children include food reactions (from eating foods to which the child is allergic, or eating too much at a time of highly seasoned foods, sweets, or fruit), "stomach flu," food poisoning, or ingestion of a poisonous or harmful nonfood substance. Drugs may be recognized as poisons by the body and rushed out in diarrhea; antibiotics upset the balance of intestinal bacteria and make loose stools more likely. Sometimes diarrhea is a reaction to emotional stress. This aspect of the child's well-being should always be considered along with the physical, especially when no other cause can be found.

WHAT A PHYSICIAN MAY DO
A physical examination will be given; this will help to assess the extent of dehydration, as will a urine specimen. Depending on the child's symptoms, the doctor may look for allergies, parasites, or infections. If a bacterial infection is discovered, antibiotics may be recommended. If the diarrhea is chronic and nothing seems to help much, a doctor might want to evaluate stool samples, do blood tests, or take X rays of the bowels. Again, before consenting, ask the reason for (and possible dangers of) each of these procedures.

WHAT YOU CAN DO AT HOME
PRACTICAL MEASURES AND NUTRITION. In order to restore the fluid lost through diarrhea, give the child generous amounts of water, vegetable juices, and broths, especially those made with barley, rice, and carrots. For infants, dilute the usual juices or formula. A liquid diet will not make diarrhea worse: it gives the intestines a chance to rest and recover normal functioning.

If the child is feeling well enough and wants to eat, start out with applesauce or grated apples, blackberries, bananas, cooked rice and barley; these foods help make the bowel movements firm again. Milk should be avoided: diarrhea can temporarily rob the body of the enzyme lactase, which is necessary for the digestion of milk sugar. Cultured milks containing lactobacillus, such as acidophilus yogurt or kefir, are usually tolerated (unless the child has a milk allergy) and improve the workings of the bowels.

Finely chop a clove of raw garlic and put it in soup or juice. (Some children will actually chew on a garlic clove). Taking 50 mg of vitamin C per hour will help when diarrhea is caused by flu.

Kaopectate (made of clay and apple pectin) can stop diarrhea; unless it is severe, however, it's best to gently replenish fluids and nutrients and let the body cleanse itself.

HERB TEAS. Peppermint, red raspberry leaf, slippery elm, comfrey, carob powder, ginger, licorice, dried blueberries, dill, fennel, cinnamon, blackberry (leaf and root).

DIARRHEA

Homeopathic Remedies.

Argentum nitricum. Diarrhea after eating too much sugar; stools may be green; pain near the groin; child may crave salt and sweets, have odd fears or worries.

Arsenicum album. Diarrhea worse after eating or cold drinks, worse at night; after spoiled food or too much fruit; child is weak, restless, chilly, afraid to be alone.

Bryonia. Diarrhea is worse in the morning, or after child becomes overheated, then drinks cold water; child feels thirsty, grumpy, irritable, wants to lie still.

Chamomilla. Hot, green, watery, slimy diarrhea with mucus; abdominal pain and gas; child is restless, whiny, angry; may have one red cheek, one pale.

China (Cinchona). Watery, frothy, putrid, yellow, or undigested stools; after fruit and milk; child has lots of gas, is chilly; may feel irritable, withdrawn, exhausted.

Colocynthis. Cutting or cramping pains in the abdomen, then diarrhea (better from doubling over or hard pressure); diarrhea after anger, emotional upset.

Gelsemium. Green or white diarrhea from excitement, nervousness, emotional upset; child looks very drowsy; may have chills up the back or flashes of heat.

Ipecacuanha. Diarrhea with extreme nausea; cutting, clutching pain, worse around the navel; stools frothy, green.

Lycopodium. Diarrhea with gas; abdomen bloated after eating, worse from 4:00 to 8:00 P.M; child may want sweets, warm drinks, be unsure of himself.

Nux vomica. Diarrhea alternates with constipation; very small amounts of brownish diarrhea pass; child is irritable, may have headache, nausea, retching.

Phosphorus. Weak, empty feeling in the abdomen; diarrhea oozes out with no control, anus feels open; child is thirsty, fearful; better from being rubbed.

Podophyllum. Diarrhea during flu or teething or after eating fruit; frequent, gushing, yellow or green, awful-smelling stools; worse in the morning and hot weather.

Pulsatilla. Queasiness with changeable diarrhea, worse at night; after eating fruit or rich food; pressure in abdomen "as from a stone"; child weepy, wants to be held.

Sulphur. Morning diarrhea; child has to leap from bed to make it to the toilet; slimy, burning, changeable diarrhea; redness and itching around the anus.

Veratrum album. Very violent, watery diarrhea; abdomen feels cold, legs weak or crampy; chill, weakness, exhaustion; child may vomit while passing stools.

ACUPRESSURE AND MASSAGE.

ST 12: A "gnawed" feeling indentation behind the upper middle of the collarbone.

ST 36: A tender point next to the outer side of the big bump at the top of the shin.

ST 25: The tender points two of the child's finger-breadths to either side of the navel.

· Massage the abdomen counterclockwise in a two-inch radius around the navel.

EAR CONDITIONS
(see also HEARING PROBLEMS)

Children's ears may give them trouble for various reasons: the most common are middle-ear infections, and blockage of the ear canal by wax, water, or foreign objects. Inflammation of the outer ear canal may also occur from fungus infection or injury; the skin of the ear canal is easily scratched and children like to poke things into it. Sometimes pain from teeth and jaws is felt in the ear. When small babies have ear problems, they can't tell you about it (except by crying), but they may pull at their ears, refuse to lie down, or move their heads in peculiar ways.

MIDDLE-EAR INFECTION (Otitis Media)
It is common for small children to develop middle-ear infections during head colds. This is partly because of the nearly horizontal position of the eustachian tubes—the passageways between throat and middle ear that regulate pressure and drainage. During a cold or infection it is easy for germs to travel from the nose and throat into the middle ear. Also, small children spend plenty of

time lying down, often with bottle or nipple in mouth; this makes introduction of foreign matter into the eustachian tubes more likely. If a tube opening is blocked by swollen lymph tissue (tonsils and adenoids swell with allergy or infection, and also grow rapidly between the ages of four and eight), a vacuum is created in the chamber behind the eardrum. Fluid or pus (which is made of white blood cells that have come in to fight the infection) then build up in the middle ear, causing pressure and pain.

Sometimes, if the eustachian tubes do not open in time to drain the middle ear, the eardrum bursts to relieve the pressure. When this happens, blood, pus, or fluid may drip out of the ear opening (sometimes seen as a crust on the child's pillow), and the pain becomes milder. Eardrum perforations are usually small tears that heal in a week or two without permanent damage; occasionally hearing may be affected, especially if bacteria have been introduced into the ear canal during misguided attempts to clean it out. With a bad infection, scar tissue may develop in the middle ear and impair hearing.

Rare but very serious complications of severe ear infections include spread of the infection to the mastoid (the bony protuberance of the skull behind the earlobe), and meningitis (spread of infection to the coverings of the brain and spinal cord). These need emergency treatment by a physician. (See MENINGITIS.)

Middle-ear infections are usually quite painful, which is awful for the parents as well as for the child. Because of the pain, and because of worry that a serious complication could result from the infection, it is hard to resist hurrying to a doctor for antibiotics. There is some evidence, however, that many ear infections treated with antibiotics do not heal any faster or with any less pain than those not treated with drugs. Also, children whose immune systems are allowed to fight off ear infections without the intervention of drugs seem to have fewer relapses and fewer later infections. Because of this, it is wise to save the use of antibiotics for cases that tend toward very dangerous complications, and otherwise try to strengthen the child's natural disease-fighting forces instead.

WHAT A PHYSICIAN MAY DO
The doctor will examine the inside of both ears and check for any signs of spreading infection or complications. Usually, if an ear in-

fection is detected or even suspected, antibiotics will be prescribed. If the infection does not seem severe, you may choose to take the written prescription but not buy the medicine unless the infection does not get better after several days of more conservative home care. Some doctors also prescribe decongestants for reducing swelling around the eustachian tubes, and antihistamines in case an allergy is involved.

If it appears that there is great pressure from infected matter in the ear, the doctor may want to perform a myringotomy (lancing of the eardrum) to relieve it.

If a child has recurrent ear infections that do not respond well to any therapy, or if there is very thick matter collecting in the middle ear, some doctors suggest the insertion of plastic tubes through the eardrums to help drain the middle ear. This is an effective solution in some cases; in others the tubes may increase infection or lead to scarring or temporary hearing loss. (Most ear infections occur at an age at which the child is learning to use and understand language; therefore even temporary hearing loss may be a learning impediment.)

WHAT YOU CAN DO AT HOME

PRACTICAL MEASURES AND NUTRITION. If the earache is very painful, fever is high, or the child seems very ill, get a medical evaluation to determine how advanced the infection is. If it is not too severe, home measures may help the child overcome it within a few days. If you choose to have your child take antibiotics, watch carefully for any signs of allergic reaction (rashes, swelling, difficulty breathing; see Emergencies in Part Two and ALLERGIES). Extra vitamins C, E, and B-complex should be given to help the body combat the drug's toxicity, and acidophilus capsules or tablets (powdered and mixed in water for infants) should be given every day during the course of medication and for two or three weeks afterward.

Make sure the child stays warm and rested and drinks plenty of fluids (broths and juices). Don't give him cow's milk during the course of the infection, even if he has no known allergy to it. Find out whether applying heat or pressure to the ear gives any comfort. Give the child as much company and amusement as possible to keep his mind off the pain.

Extra vitamins A, C, E, and zinc will help fight infection.

NATURAL APPLICATIONS. Lukewarm olive oil with mullein and/or garlic steeped in it is an old and often effective natural remedy; dropped gently into an aching ear (or saturating a piece of cotton with it and placing it in the ear canal), it can soothe the ear and draw out infection. However, it is important that you know how severe an infection is before using eardrops of any kind. If the eardrum is perforated or about to burst, the oil may carry bacteria into the middle ear and make the infection worse.

Poultices made of a clove of garlic (or the center of an onion), boiled, cooled, and laid across the aching ear (*not* pushed inside it) and bound on with cloth, can help—if the child will keep them on. These should be changed every day.

HERB TEAS. Echinacea, calendula, red clover.

HOMEOPATHIC REMEDIES.

Ferrum phosphoricum. When an earache is just beginning; outer ear red, eardrum red and bulging; child flushed, tired or restless, in good spirits when pain abates.

Aconitum napellus. Sudden, hot, throbbing, cutting pain, after exposure to cold or wind; worse at night; child is fearful, agitated. Another remedy may follow this one.

Belladonna. Bouts of earache come and go suddenly; child is restless, or in a stupor; hot, flushed, pounding pulse; worse from jarring and motion.

Chamomilla. Pains come in waves that seem intolerable; child is extremely irritable or angry, though he wants to be carried; one or both cheeks may be red; worse from heat and wind.

Hepar sulphuris calcareum. Infection is advanced, with pus in the middle ear; sticking pains; child can't stand to have the ear touched; is extremely sensitive to drafts, acts angry.

Magnesia phosphorica. Severe ache, mostly nerve pain; worse from cold; better from heat and pressure.

Mercurius vivus. Advanced infection, shooting pain, roaring in ears; swollen face and lymph nodes; pain worse at night and from any change in temperature; child sweats, drools in sleep, has puffy tongue, bad breath.

Pulsatilla. Ear is swollen, hot, red; chronic infections, deep itching in the ear; child is weepy, clinging, is not thirsty, dislikes warmth and wants fresh air.

ACUPRESSURE AND MASSAGE. (See also INFECTIONS.) Unless it really bothers the child, gentle massage of the neck muscles (front and back), the points around and behind the ear, and the ear itself, will help to drain the lymphatic tissues and relieve congestion and pain.

OUTER EAR INFECTION (Otitis Externa)

When the sensitive skin of the outer-ear canal becomes infected by bacteria, it can be extremely painful. Pulling the ear, lying on it, or moving it in any way may hurt, and redness, swelling, or discharge can usually be seen. Ear-canal infection is often caused when a scratch is made in the ear canal by sticking something into it to scratch or clear out wax. Sometimes a boil forms in the ear. When a child swims or is in the water a lot (especially dirty water), fungus may take hold in the skin of the ear canal; this may look gray or whitish and be itchy and painful. If the skin of the outer ear is red and swollen, or the inflammation seems to be rapidly spreading to other areas, check with a doctor right away.

WHAT A PHYSICIAN MAY DO

A doctor will examine the ear canal and surrounding area to check for the extent of infection or complications (hard, inflamed lymph nodes or simultaneous middle-ear infections). The canal will be cleaned, and antibiotic or antifungal drops or ointment prescribed.

WHAT YOU CAN DO AT HOME

The canal may be very gently cleaned by placing a piece of gauze or cotton soaked in clean water, then dipped in apple-cider vinegar, inside the canal. This will change the acidity of the skin and help the infection heal. After eight hours, the cotton may be removed, and vinegar diluted 3:1 with water dabbed along the canal with a cotton swab several times a day. Echinacea or goldenseal tinctures, diluted 5:1, may be used in the same way.

IMPACTED EARWAX

Sometimes earwax is very dry or sticky and does not move naturally out of the ear canal. It may have been pushed back toward the eardrum during attempts to clean it out by sticking a swab (or a pen, or anything) into the ear. When the canal is clogged by wax, hearing is affected and the skin inside the canal may be itchy or uncomfortable.

WHAT A PHYSICIAN MAY DO
After making sure there is no middle-ear infection and the eardrum is intact, a doctor may loosen the wax by irrigating the ear with a special syringe and a tepid antiseptic solution, or may remove the impacted wax with a special spoon.

WHAT YOU CAN DO AT HOME
Have the child sit in a hot bathtub for a while, to liquefy the wax, then wipe it out of the outer hole with a washcloth. Massaging the fleshy part of the ear, and points in front and behind, helps to loosen wax.

If the ear is not infected or injured in any way, the wax may be dissolved by dropping a solution of half hydrogen peroxide and half tepid water into the ear. Have the child hold his head to the side (full ear side up) for several minutes, then to the other side to let the loosened wax trickle out. This should be done daily for about a week. Never introduce anything very cold or hot into the ear; this can cause dizziness and nausea.

ECZEMA

Any rash that reddens, inflames, dries, or forms scales, crusts, bumps, or blisters on the skin is eczema, but the term is usually used to refer to the chronic allergic form known as *atopic dermatitis.* The rash may occur on the cheeks, eyelids, scalp, wrists, backs of the upper arms, or inner surface of the elbows and knees. Eczema occurs most often in families with a history of asthma, hay fever, and other allergic disorders. Emotional stress, sweating, drying forms of indoor heat, changes in temperature and humidity, food allergy, and contact with irritating substances such as wool, synthetic fabrics, or certain laundry detergents, lotions, and medicines, often make it worse. Scratching may further irritate the skin and make a secondary bacterial infection more likely.

WHAT A PHYSICIAN MAY DO

A doctor, depending on her opinions and training, will either try to protect and strengthen the child's system against the underlying allergic condition, or will attempt to suppress the symptoms of the rash by use of drugs like antihistamines and corticosteroid ointments. After the use of antihistamines, allergic rashes often return and may become chronic. Corticosterioid drugs, absorbed through the broken skin, can upset the balance of hormones in the child's growing body and derange immune response, creating problems much worse than eczema.

WHAT YOU CAN DO AT HOME

PRACTICAL MEASURES. Any underlying allergies should be detected and treated. (See ALLERGIES.) The child's skin should be kept clean with plain water, avoiding soap and bubble bath. Keep the child's fingernails short and clean to prevent injury from scratching and reduce the chance of bacterial infection. Swimming in the ocean (where it is not polluted) and exposing skin to moderate sunlight and fresh air are beneficial.

Medicated greases and lotions, especially those containing perfumes or colorings, may make the skin condition worse and keep air away from the rash, increasing the time it takes to heal. To slightly lubricate the skin and protect it from rubbing and irritation, rub in a little olive oil or lanolin-based cream containing vitamins E and A, aloe vera gel, or calendula lotion. After bathing, rub cucumber juice on the skin or dab apple-cider vinegar, calendula ointment, or cooled teas of elder flower, blackberry leaf, goldenseal, or yellow dock on the areas of rash. Oatmeal, moistened and wrapped in a cloth that is held on the irritated areas, will help soothe the itching.

NUTRITION. A diet that emphasizes fresh raw vegetables and fruits (cucumbers and watercress are especially good) and is low in animal products and salt can improve metabolism and help the child's body eliminate toxins. The child should not eat refined, fried, or processed foods, sugar, strong spices, or beef. Kelp, lecithin, whey powder, flaxseed oil, and brewer's yeast are helpful. Essential fatty acids should be consumed in the form of cold-pressed oils such as sunflower, olive, and sesame. Extra vitamins A,

C, E, balanced B-complex including PABA, zinc, omega-3 fatty acids, and a multivitamin and mineral supplement should be taken every day.

HOMEOPATHIC REMEDIES. A constitutional remedy is the proper approach for dealing with eczema. See an experienced homeopathic prescriber.

For acupressure and massage, see ALLERGIES.

EYE CONDITIONS

Clues to a child's health—mental, emotional, and physical—are often given by his eyes: both in the way he looks out of them and the way they appear to you when you are looking in. Eyes that are dull, or too bright, may tell you that the child is agitated, feverish, or ill. Eyes that don't focus may signify poisoning, confusion, distraction, head injury, or nearsightedness. Puffy, reddened eyes can mean infection, irritation, allergy, or recent crying.

Since vision is the eyes' main function, any condition involving the eyes can interfere with a child's comfort and clarity of mind. From the moment of birth, (except in cases altered by the use of anesthetics), a baby is seeing in varying stages of acuity and learning from what he sees.

In many older children, headaches, so-called learning problems, and short attention span are eventually found to be the result of poor or distorted vision; behavior problems and headaches from schoolwork may stem from strain on the eye muscles and the frustration of trying to see with eyes that aren't working properly. Sometimes visual problems are hard to detect. If a child has been nearsighted all her life, for instance, she may not be aware that the marks on the blackboard aren't buglike smudges to everyone, or that trees have visible leaves and twigs even from a distance, not just when you put your nose up to them.

Some eye problems are detected by the simple eye tests given in schools, but children who have used cleverness all their lives to compensate for inadequate eyesight, or children whose problems are not near- or farsightedness but some sort of distortion (such as astigmatism), may pass these tests and still be burdened by problems in perception.

Other common eye problems, which may or may not interfere with vision, are caused by infections, irritations, and injuries to the eyes, or may be part of a disorder involving other parts of the body, such as measles, allergy, head injury, or seizures.

Eye symptoms that require prompt medical attention include: any loss or lasting abnormality of vision; any severe eye pain, or eye pain caused by exposure to light; pupils that appear unequal or irregularly shaped; extreme redness, especially if it surrounds the iris; bleeding; serious injury; and a foreign object or chemical in the eye.

FOREIGN SUBSTANCES IN THE EYE

If any stinging or burning substance gets into a child's eye, flush it out with pure water immediately. Most shampoos and soaps do little more than irritate the eye tissues temporarily, but there may be dangerous chemicals in household substances (cleaning fluids, insecticides, disinfectants, cosmetics) that a curious or careless child may get in his eyes.

The child should be rushed to the sink or hose and the eye(s) held open under a mild stream of water, or doused with an eyecup (a small cup that fits snugly over the eye while the head is tipped back; these can be bought at drugstores). Hold his head so the water washes the eyeball from many different angles, to be sure all areas are washed out. Do this for at least fifteen minutes, or until the stinging is gone. There may be a bit of unpleasant sensation remaining afterwards, just from the water. (If there is not water available, you should repeatedly lick inside the child's eye, and spit out the irritating substance.) After this, telephone a poison control center or doctor to find out how dangerous the substance is and whether more treatment may be needed. If pain remains or increases, get professional help right away.

FOREIGN OBJECTS IN THE EYE

Children walking in the wind or playing outdoors often get specks of dirt or sand in their eyes. These are readily washed out by tears or rinsed away with water. The white of the eye may be reddened afterwards, and the sensation of something in the eye may linger because of scratching or irritation of the conjunctiva (the outer lining of the eyeball and eyelids) or the cornea (the sturdier, clear covering of the eye). Sometimes, however, the offending substance—for instance, a tiny splinter of glass or metal—cannot be flushed out and, visible or not, can cause constant discomfort and eventually lead to infection, damage to the eye structures, or even loss of sight.

WHAT A PHYSICIAN MAY DO

A doctor will examine the eye and inner lids. A fluorescent dye may be applied and the eye examined under ultraviolet light for scratches or punctures in the covering of the eye. A foreign body may be removed with an eyewash, a cotton swab, a small needle, or magnet. If this is not enough to take care of it, a general practitioner may call on an eye surgeon or ophthalmologist for special help.

WHAT YOU CAN DO AT HOME

Holding the lids apart, let a mild stream of tap water run over the eyeball from several angles, to reach all corners. Or gently wash out the eye with an eyecup. Inspect the eye carefully, in good light, from the front and from each side. If you see a speck or splinter, try to remove it gently with a damp wisp of cotton. If it seems to be stuck in the eye, especially if it seems to have penetrated the globe, or if there is blood, get an expert's help. Removing the object with forceps or a swab may be a simple operation, but a worried, squirming child, unless firmly immobilized, is at risk of serious injury from being poked by the instruments.

If you don't find anything in the eye, pull the lids slightly outward and move them up, down, and to the sides to try to dislodge any trapped particles, then flush with water again. Sometimes a drop of lukewarm milk introduced into the eye will isolate the foreign material and soothe the irritation.

If you still find nothing, and the pain is not so severe that the child can't be distracted, cover the eye with an eyepatch (a few layers of gauze taped on in a way that is not too bothersome). This will discourage further irritation, both from use and from rubbing. If the eye is not better within forty-eight hours, get professional help.

INJURY TO THE EYE

When a child's eye is poked by an object like a stick, fingernail, or wire, it is wise to be sure that no deeper structure has been hurt. With even a minor scratch of superficial tissues, the child may cry and be upset for a while, but if the pain lasts for more than a few minutes and the child has difficulty keeping the eye open, the cornea may have been scratched.

A scratch on the cornea is very painful and takes time to heal. Not much can be done but to cover the eye with an eyepatch (or fold gauze in several layers and tape it on comfortably) and wait. Still, it is good to have the counsel of a doctor who will help you watch for complications. If the scratch is serious, an antibiotic may be applied to avoid infection. If the scratch is minor, a poultice of grated apple wrapped in a clean, damp cotton cloth and left on for an hour or so will help.

A hard blow or other serious trauma to the globe of the eye may damage delicate structures inside the eye, dislocate the lens, and cause hemorrhage or fluid leakage, and needs the attention of an ophthalmologist. The homeopathic remedy *Symphytum* is often useful in cases of trauma to the eyeball.

CROSSED EYES (Strabismus)

This condition occurs when the muscles that control eye position and movement are not working properly and the eyes do not function in coordination. When this happens, the brain receives visual messages from each eye separately, but soon discounts the information it receives from the turned-in, "lazy" eye.

In babies six months of age or younger, a slightly cross-eyed appearance is normal. The eye muscles have not yet learned to coordinate eye position. Also, there are often skin folds on the inner corners of an infant's eyes that make the eyes appear crossed when actually they are not.

In an older child, you can check for crossed eyes by having her gaze straight ahead in good light and cover, then uncover, first one eye, then the other. Notice the eye positions: each eye should remain coordinated with the other and not drift off. Another way of testing this is to move an object slowly past the child's eyes, from one side to the other, and see if both eyes follow it together.

Crossed or "lazy" eyes that are detected early are often

easily corrected, since the eye muscles haven't been too long accustomed to working the wrong way. A number of cases have been overcome by use of eye exercises, eyepatches, special glasses, applied kinesiology, cross-crawl therapy, acupuncture, and correction of spinal or cranial misalignments by specially trained chiropractors or osteopaths.

When these measures do not succeed, surgery is sometimes recommended to tighten or loosen various muscles attached to the eyeball. It is important for parents to understand that any surgery, however simple, may be a risk to a child's life. It is not unknown for children undergoing operations for minor problems to die from improper anesthesia. Since surgery for strabismus artificially alters the delicate eye muscles, measures for restoring normal neurological and muscular balance should be thoroughly explored first; there are cases where a later balance restoration has left the child's eyes crossed *because of* the operation.

SWELLING AROUND THE EYES

The tissue around the eyes is very loose and therefore susceptible to swelling. Allergy, fatigue, crying, respiratory infections, bug bites, or injuries are common causes of swelling. A compress of warm parsley tea left on for several minutes may help relieve puffiness.

If the eye area has been injured by a blow, applying a cold damp cloth, ice pack, or poultice for five or ten minutes will reduce the amount of bruising and swelling and lessen the discomfort (and drama) of the subsequent black eye.

Occasionally the tissue around the eyes may become swollen because of a more serious disorder, such as trouble with liver or kidney function; however, if this is the case, the child will also show swelling of other parts of the body (wrists, ankles, abdomen), as well as other symptoms of illness.

BLOCKED TEAR DUCTS

It is not uncommon for the ducts that drain tears from an infant's eyes to become blocked, making the eyes water in excess and be sticky. This condition can usually be relieved by using warm, moist compresses on the eye, and gently massaging the skin downward from the inner corner of the eye toward the nose. If there is no redness or infection, this may be done for several months and the duct will eventually be cleared. A doctor should be consulted if infection occurs. (See also CONJUNCTIVITIS, below.)

STYES

Styes are little boils or pimples on the edge of the eyelid, usually caused by bacterial (staphylococcal) infection of the oil or sweat glands. Styes are sometimes painful but usually not serious and heal within a day or two. Applying a warm, wet washcloth to the eye for fifteen or twenty minutes several times a day will usually make them drain or heal. (Parsley tea may be used instead of water.) Dabbing on calendula lotion (one drop of tincture in a teaspoonful of water) may help. If the stye does not get well, is on the inside of the eyelid, turns into a hard red bump, or is accompanied by a feeling of sickness, get advice from a physician.

For homeopathic remedies, see CONJUNCTIVITIS, below.

CONJUNCTIVITIS (Pinkeye)

This is an inflamed condition of the conjunctiva, the membrane that covers the whites of the eye and lines the insides of the lid. The symptoms are redness, burning, itching, and a discharge of mucus or pus that may glue the eyelids shut. The cause is usually viral, especially if accompanied by swollen lymph nodes and cold symptoms, sore throat, or fever. If bacterial, the discharge will be thick and greenish-yellow.

Conjunctivitis may also be caused by measles, allergy, irritation from chemicals or environmental pollutants (fumes from traffic or from factories, woodsmoke, cigarette smoke, contaminated water, swimming pool chlorine), dust irritation, windburn, or sunburn. In newborn babies, conjunctivitis may result from the silver nitrate or antibiotic eyedrops that are given as a matter of course in many hospitals for prevention of gonorrheal infection.

WHAT A PHYSICIAN MAY DO

A doctor will inspect the eyes and possibly take a culture sample of discharge. She may clean the eyes with an eyewash solution, or teach you to do it.

If the problem is a bacterial infection, antibiotic eyedrops may be recommended. If the cause is allergic, antihistamines or cortisone drops may be prescribed. It is best to avoid these medicines, as they may make the problem rebound—that is, the symptoms may leave, but then, when the drug is through suppressing them, come bounding back. In certain cases, such as herpes simplex infection, the wrong choice of medicine makes the condition much worse.

WHAT YOU CAN DO AT HOME

PRACTICAL MEASURES AND NATURAL APPLICATIONS. Pinkeye is contagious, so care should be taken that no one else uses towels, pillowcases, or washcloths that have been touched by the pinkeye patient; after use they should all be carefully washed.

Wet a piece of clean cotton with sterile water (boiled and cooled) and apply it to the eyelid edges to soften and wipe away the crusts. A poultice of grated apple laid directly on the eye and covered with a clean, damp cotton cloth for half an hour several times a day is soothing and draws out infection. Potato, cucumber, goat's-milk yogurt, or violet leaves also make effective poultices.

Eyewashes can be made from one drop fresh lemon juice in an ounce of pure water; or alfalfa, orange peel, chamomile, or eyebright steeped in boiling water, then cooled. Eyewash from an infusion of goldenseal is good for bacterial infection.

Viral pinkeye usually clears itself in a couple of days, so all that is needed is cleanliness and waiting. If bacterial pinkeye doesn't improve within a week or gets worse, check with a doctor for a different course of treatment.

If the irritation is caused by allergy, try to identify the allergic agent. If it is an air pollutant or pollen, it may be best to keep the child indoors, or have her wear special protective glasses to keep her eyes from being exposed too much.

Over-the-counter drops for soothing the eyes sometimes contain toxic substances and are not recommended for children.

NUTRITION. During any sort of eye problem, the diet should be fortified with vitamins A, C and B-complex. Taking 100 mg of vitamin C every hour is helpful in the case of viral or bacterial infection. Carrots and carrot juice, apples, potatoes, cucumbers, sprouted seeds and grains, watercress, goat's-milk yogurt, and brewer's yeast are good additions to the diet.

HOMEOPATHIC REMEDIES.

Apis mellifica. Watery, puffy swelling; eyelids stick together; burning, stinging pain relieved by application of cold water.

Argentum nitricum. Advanced infection with pus formation; swelling and redness of the whites of the eyes and the inner corners; worse from light and a warm room; better from cold, fresh air, cold water.

Euphrasia. Chronic itching and inflammation, accompanied by headache and constant runny nose; burning tears make the cheeks look varnished.

Hepar sulphuris calcareum. Eyelids feel sore and bruised; eyes feel pulled back into the head, with burning pain; better from warm applications; chronic styes.

Natrum muriaticum. Swollen eyelids, tears burn, eyes feel bruised; discharge of mucus or pus; child seems to need consolation but may refuse it.

Pulsatilla. Conjunctivitis with a cold or measles; thick, yellow discharge; styes on lower lids; worse in the morning; itching, sensitive; better from open air.

Rhus toxicodendron. Inflammation of the inner surface of the eyelids; intense pain on moving or touching the eyes; spasm of eyelids; thick yellow discharge; worse after midnight; better from warmth.

Sulphur. Intense smarting and itching with sticking pains; hot tears; eyes bloodshot; lids are contracted in the morning; child can't look at light.

ACUPRESSURE AND MASSAGE.

LV 3: A tender point midway between the first and second metatarsal bones.

· Massage the earlobe and the inside of the knuckle closest to the thumbnail.

· Massage all tender points on the bony ridge around the eye socket.

FEET AND LEGS

The following conditions are occasionally seen in growing children as the skeletal structure develops. They are usually not serious, and the child will grow into his or her frame as muscular development catches up.

FLAT FEET
Babies often appear to have very flat feet. This is not a structural abnormality but a normal fat pad on the sole that prevents the arch from showing. As a child learns to walk, the arches become more

distinct with muscle use and development. If, however, a bone seems to protrude from a baby's foot in an odd place, or if the two feet do not look alike, it is wise to have this checked.

ARCH PROBLEMS

When an older child reports pain in his feet, or if the heels of his shoes wear out on the inner edge, it may be that his arches are not in proper alignment. Often such a problem is the result of badly fitting shoes, but the bones of the feet (or legs, pelvis, or spine) may need to be adjusted by a qualified podiatrist, chiropodist, or chiropractor.

BOWLEGS

Most infants and toddlers up to age two show some bowing of the legs that disappears when the ankles are touched together. If a gap of more than one and a half inches shows in an older child standing with the ankles touching, keep track of the gap over weeks and months. If it increases you may want to consult a doctor who works in noninvasive ways with extremities.

KNOCK-KNEES

This condition is often accompanied by "pigeon toes," as the toes turn in to help with balance. This is usually seen between the ages of three and six, and goes away with time. Measure the gap between the ankles, with the knees touching; if, after age six, the gap is wider than two inches, keep track of it. If it enlarges, you may want to consult a physician.

CONGENITAL HIP DISLOCATION

This is usually detected at birth, or before the age of one. Its cause is not entirely clear, but seems to involve lax ligaments and muscle spasms that prevent the hip joint from staying stable. When the child is lying down with the legs bent at both knee and hip, then opened outward, a click may be heard coming from one or both hips; sometimes the child's thigh cannot be touched to the surface on which she is lying. If the condition is present on only one side, one leg may look oddly bent or shorter than the other, or the skin creases of the two thighs may not look alike. Having the child ride on the mother's back or hip, or wearing thick padded diapers or splints to keep the knees high and widely spaced, will help hold the hips in proper position while the muscles and ligaments develop. A children's orthopedist can advise patients in home treatment. In extreme cases, surgery must be performed.

CLUBFOOT (Talipes)
Usually seen at birth, this sort of deformity may occur in different positions. Treatment consists of massaging and moving the foot toward the correct position, several times a day. Clubfoot may also be treated through taping, casting, or corrective shoes.

GENERAL POSITIONAL ABNORMALITIES
Many foot and leg problems are actually the result of improper alignment of other body structures, such as the spine, pelvis, and related muscles. If, when the child is lying on her back, one or both feet cannot be turned outward, it may be that the leg is related to the hip at an incorrect angle. If, while the child is sitting on a table, the outer anklebone is seen to be in front of the inner one, one of the lower bones of the leg may not be correctly positioned. If the muscles of the legs are weak or hurt, there may be a spinal misalignment. In these situations, specific exercises and *gentle* manipulations from a chiropractor or osteopath may correct the problem.

Sometimes a malformation of a bone or joint can cause bones to be (or appear to be) out of position, so that posture or walking are impaired. In this case, consult a children's orthopedist.

WHAT A PHYSICIAN MAY DO
An examination will be made of the way the child walks and stands, and of the joints and shape of the hips, back, and legs. Measurements and comparisons between the two sides of the body will probably be made. If a bone or joint problem is suspected, X rays may be taken to help make a more specific diagnosis. If the problem is painful or seriously impairs the child's motion, X rays may be justified. A pediatrician or general practitioner may suggest that you take your child to an orthopedic specialist; these doctors often apply splints or braces, or recommend surgery. Surgery is usually not recommended before the age of eight or nine unless the problems are very severe, because children so often grow out of them.

Well-meaning as they may be, many orthopedists and MDs

do not realize that the manipulative techniques used by chiropractors and other natural health practitioners are often successful in correcting orthopedic problems. If an orthopedic surgeon's services are recommended, it may be worthwhile to talk to other types of physicians, too. Be sure to choose a practitioner who is competent, extremely gentle, and accustomed to treating children. Very low-force techniques of manipulation cause no damage and can work just as well or better than the vigorous ones.

WHAT YOU CAN DO AT HOME

PRACTICAL MEASURES. Make sure your child spends part of each day in physical exercise: running and playing are great, unless they cause pain during the activity or later. Swimming and bicycling are excellent non–weight-bearing activities that exercise the muscles without placing stress on bones and joints. Make sure the child's shoes are comfortable, well-cushioned, and fit properly; let her go barefoot at times in safe, clean places. Try to discourage sleeping on the stomach, as this encourages toeing-in and adds extra stress to the spine.

NUTRITION. Dietary deficiencies may contribute to leg and foot conditions. Even if the tendency is hereditary, good nutrition may help. Sufficient protein, calcium, magnesium, vitamins A, D, C, E, and B-complex are necessary for proper growth and healthy bones in a child. Many bone problems improve remarkably once vitamin D is added to a deficient child's diet. Vitamin D is needed for proper metabolism of minerals and the way they are deposited in bones; however, vitamin D should not be supplied in too great amounts, as it accumulates in the body, and overdose is toxic. Synthetic vitamin D (D_2, calciferol) is chemically different from the natural form (D_3, activated ergosterol) and is not really what the body is designed to use. Fish oil is a good source of Vitamin D_3, but regular, moderate sunshine (if available) is the best. Sunshine converts a substance in skin oil into natural vitamin D; because of this, it is better not to scrub too frequently with soap. Use plain warm water except when the child is especially dirty, and have him bathe after, not before, he goes out to play in the sun.

HOMEOPATHIC REMEDIES. If a child has a serious developmental condition, a constitutional remedy chosen by a trained prescriber will be more helpful than symptomatic treatment. Remedies often used to help with bone growth and development include:

Calcarea carbonica. Child is late in walking and teething, with tendency to swollen lymph nodes and weak bones; sweats on exertion and in sleep; flabby, chilly, easily tired, poorly coordinated; craves eggs and sweets; afraid of the dark (may "see" faces); worse in cold, damp weather; better from warmth and lying down.

Calcarea phosphorica. Stiff, sore legs that may feel cold and numb, tired from walking; frequent headaches; complaining, forgetful child who always wants to "go somewhere"; craves bacon, ham, junk food; may have food allergies.

Phosphorus. Child is thin, with narrow chest; inclined toward chest colds, nosebleeds; excitable and talkative but easily tired; face flushes easily; craves salt, cold drinks, ice cream; bright, talkative, imaginative; strong fears, likes company.

Silicea. Child is thin, undernourished-looking, with a large head; soft teeth, bones; nails ridged or have white spots; easily tired; conscientious, easily embarrassed; head feels cold, frequent headaches, likes to wear hats; sweaty head, offensive sweat from feet.

ACUPRESSURE AND MASSAGE.

BL 11: The points in the muscles two of the child's thumb-widths to the sides of the vertebra below the bony bump at the base of the neck.

KI 1: A point on the sole between the pads on the ball of the foot.

KI 3: The tender point just behind the upper rear aspect of the inner anklebone.

FEVER

Most people accept the figure 98.6 degrees F. as the normal body temperature. However, like most other traits of human beings, a healthy temperature varies from occasion to occasion and from individual to individual. Children's temperatures may drop or rise three or four degrees during a day when they are not in the least ill. Generally, fever is a temperature greater than 105°.

The ability to create fever when an infection threatens is one of the body's most valuable talents. During a fever, the body temperature rises and the activity and efficiency of disease-fighting

elements in the immune system are increased; thus the body becomes an unfavorable environment for the survival of many
disease-associated microorganisms. Because fever occurs in illness, and illness is uncomfortable, many parents think that bringing down the temperature artifically will help the child get better
faster. Actually, reducing a moderate fever (lower than 103 degrees) may slow the healing process: an elevated temperature is a
welcome sign that the immune system is doing its job.

The height of a fever does not necessarily reflect the severity
of the illness. Some mild viral infections can take the temperature
up to 105; some more serious diseases (appendicitis, for example)
may raise it only to 101. Most children's fevers are part of viral or
bacterial infections like cold, flu, ear infection, sore throat, roseola, measles, and chicken pox. Serious diseases accompanied by
fever—such as kidney infections, pneumonia, meningitis, and encephalitis—occur more rarely, but when they do a doctor's help is
needed. Other symptoms than fever should carry more weight in
assessing how ill a child is. How sick he *seems*—how uncomfortable or debilitated he is, how much appetite and energy he has—
is a better indication than the reading on a thermometer.

Shivering often occurs alternately with fever. Chills are actually a manifestation of fever, a reaction to the difference between
the temperatures inside and outside the body. Sweating is usually a
sign that a fever is breaking and about to go down. Each child has
his own way of reacting to high fevers—some seem only slightly
sick, some talk irrationally, or talk or walk in their sleep, some cry
or are easily startled, some shudder or have a convulsion (see CON-
VULSIONS). Once you are used to your child's reaction, you can
more easily determine which symptoms require extra concern
and which do not.

Any fever in a child younger than four months old, any fever
that lasts more than twenty-four hours in a child less than one year
old, any fever that has not improved at all within three days or has
lasted more than a week, and any fever of 105 or higher should receive a doctor's attention.

If you are worried or unsure about a child's fever and illness,
call a doctor and describe the symptoms. Observe the child carefully before you call so you'll have accurate information. Try to
find a doctor who will discuss the child's condition over the
phone; it is not always in the best interests of a feverish child to

take him out in the night or in foul weather to a doctor's office or emergency room.

WHAT A PHYSICIAN MAY DO

A doctor will try to determine the cause of the fever and treat that. Very high temperature will be controlled, with some of the same techniques you might use at home. For very rapidly rising fevers, a doctor may use ice-water baths or ice packs—during which the child's temperature must be monitored carefully to prevent shock or hypothermia. Acetaminophen, and occasionally aspirin, are used to lower the temperature; most other antifever drugs are even more dangerous.

WHAT YOU CAN DO AT HOME

PRACTICAL MEASURES. Take the child's temperature when he feels very hot to the touch or seems to be ill or listless. Unless he seems very sick or has a tendency toward febrile seizures, there is no need to constantly monitor the fever, since the reading on the thermometer in itself is less significant than other symptoms. The easiest way to take a child's temperature is to raise his arm and place the thermometer bulb snugly in his armpit, then lower the arm and keep it close to his side for three or four minutes. Hold him on your lap or sit beside him and calmly read a story or talk until the time is up. Axillary (armpit) temperature readings are usually about half a degree lower than oral, and rectal readings one degree higher (i.e., if the child's oral "normal" is 98.6 degrees F., his axillary "normal" would be close to 98, the rectal 99.6). If you choose to take the temperature orally or rectally for slightly more accurate readings, remember that a child younger than four cannot be expected to keep a thermometer in his mouth without biting it. Rectal temperatures (using a round-bulbed rectal thermometer) should only be taken in children under four, and then only if they are not embarrassed or upset by the process. Plastic stick-on strips are also available that take temperature readings from the forehead.

Simple, safe ways of easing the discomfort of a fever can be found by paying attention to what the child wants. If he's feeling too hot, extra clothing and covers can be removed; usually a sheet is enough covering, unless the room is much too cold. If the child begins to feel chilly, covers should be used, then taken off again when he warms up.

If the fever is high and the child needs some relief, use natural, drugless ways of bringing it down. A warm bath (96 degrees F. or so) is still lower than normal body temperature, so it can cool a feverish child. Sponging of the arms, legs, and face with a cloth dampened with water or mint tea will cool the surface of the body by evaporation and make the child more comfortable. Do not use alcohol; its fumes should not be inhaled. Soaking the feet in a basin of cool mint tea can also help.

When chills are caused by fever, make the child feel just warm enough to be comfortable. This does not mean bundling him up in ten blankets and turning up the furnace (unless the room is very cold), as these methods may drive the internal fever higher. However, if one extra blanket, or cuddling up with someone, or having something warm to drink makes the child feel cozier, use them. Sometimes letting a child sit in a bathtub of tepid water (about 90–95 degrees) will help, since it may make the child's skin feel warmer without increasing the fever.

Aspirin or acetaminophen is often routinely used for bringing down fevers over 100 degrees. It is true that these medicines slightly reduce discomfort, but the fact that they are working against the body's natural means of fighting infection, and may in this way be lowering the child's resistance and making the illness last longer, should give parents food for thought. These medicines, especially in sensitive individuals or in certain illnesses, can be very dangerous.

NUTRITION. A child should not eat during an active fever but should be given lots of extra liquid: juices, herb teas, broths, or water. Some prefer frozen fruit juice or ice cubes to suck on. Fluids are very important to prevent dehydration. Extra vitamins A, C, E, B-complex, and zinc help fight infection.

HERB TEAS. Calendula, dandelion, gentian, yerba santé.

HOMEOPATHIC REMEDIES.
 Aconitum napellus. Fever comes on very suddenly and intensely; pounding pulse; dry, burning skin; child is frightened, thirsty; worse at evening and night.

Arsenicum album. Fever with hot head and chills; burning pains are relieved by heat; child is restless and fearful but also weak; thirsty, drinks in sips.

Belladonna. Sudden, high fever; child is hot, red-faced, excitable, with dilated glassy eyes, may be delirious.

Ferrum phosphoricum. Moderate fever, child is flushed, has red cheeks, and may be irritable; cold applications help. Useful at the start of any inflammatory illness.

Gelsemium. Fever with aching, drowsiness, heavy limbs, chills along the spine; child is usually not thirsty; eyes look droopy.

Phosphorus. Chills and fever; sweats in sleep; child may be fearful, or alert and cheerful despite very high temperature; likes to be rubbed; thirsty for cold drinks.

Pulsatilla. Fever with chilliness in child who is usually warm-blooded; child is changeable, tearful, clinging; worse at night, in stuffy room, or after eating.

ACUPRESSURE AND MASSAGE.

LI 4: The point at the end of the crease between the thumb and index finger.

ST 12: A "gnawed" feeling indentation behind the upper middle of the collarbone.

SP 6: A tender point three of the child's finger-breadths above the inner anklebone.

ST 36: A tender point next to the outer side of the big bump at the top of the shin.

LI 11: A tender point at the thumb-side end of the elbow-crease when the arm is bent.

FINGERNAILS AND TOENAILS

Children's nails most commonly need attention because of dirtiness, length, or injury, but may require extra care in conditions caused by infection, bad hygiene, or improper growth. Some children have nails that grow very slowly, are flimsy and peeling, or are brittle with a tendency to split. This may signify a lack in the diet of good-quality protein and/or the mineral silicon—raw vegetables and oats are good sources of this element. Ridges and white spots on the nails often indicate mineral deficiencies, particularly of zinc. It is normal for very small infants to have weak or almost nonexistent nails.

Most children don't like having their nails cut, and some even claim that it hurts. This may be due to their uncertainty about *any* part of their bodies being cut; it may also be that in the past their nails have been cut uncomfortably short; or it may be that it actually does hurt—some people have very sensitive fingertips. Children may prefer the use of fingernail clippers to scissors. Try to cut the nails short, but leave a tiny ridge of white to shield the tender skin.

If a small child has an itching skin condition such as eczema, sunburn, or chicken pox, it is important that the nails be kept very short and clean so that bacteria are not introduced by scratching.

SMASHED FINGERTIP OR TOE

The tips of fingers and toes are well supplied with nerves, which means that a finger caught in a door, or a stubbed toe, can be exquisitely painful without serious damage having been done. If the pain does not lessen after half an hour or so, it would be wise to have the injury examined.

You should look carefully at the finger or toe, in case it has become misshapen (as from a fracture) or is badly cut or the nail is torn. If there appears to be any serious injury, go for medical help as soon as possible. Remember, if surgery seems likely, an anesthetic may be necessary, so you should not give the child anything to eat or drink.

WHAT A PHYSICIAN MAY DO

An X ray may be taken if a fracture is suspected. In fingertip or toe-tip injuries, special treatment is usually needed only for fractures involving the joint. Any cuts or tears that require repair will be taken care of. If the pain is intense or infection likely, pain-killers or antibiotic ointments may be prescribed.

WHAT YOU CAN DO AT HOME

Immediately apply an ice pack, or hold the hurt part under cold running water for five or ten minutes. This will slow the swelling and lessen the pain. The homeopathic remedy *Hypericum* is best for injury to body parts with many nerves, with excessive pain; the remedy *Arnica* is used for any kind of bruising.

If blood or fluid collected under a smashed nail causes pain and pressure, you can carefully melt a hole in the nail to relieve it. Hold a straightened paper clip with a pair of pliers and heat the end in a flame, then gently touch it to the nail until a small hole is melted. Do this in the middle of the discolored portion, which will be full of collected fluid. The child will not feel the tip, as long as you're careful. If you (or your child) feel too squeamish about this, have a doctor do it.

INFECTIONS OF THE NAILS

Infection of nails can begin when a cut or hangnail or chronic irritation allows entry of a microorganism (such as Pseudomonas or Candida albicans) or fungus (such as ringworm or athlete's foot). The nails may look dull and become thick or loosened, the skin may become red and tender, crack or peel, and pus or dirty-looking matter may appear around the edges. If the finger or toe is very inflamed, hot, or throbbing, and does not improve with natural treatments within a day or two—or if the child feels ill—a doctor should be consulted.

WHAT A PHYSICIAN MAY DO

Scrapings of skin may be examined under a microscope, or a culture made from them. Over-the-counter ointments or powders (with antibiotics for bacterial infections, nystatin for Candida, salicylic or undecylenic acid for fungus) may be suggested. If these do not work, stronger prescription medicines may be tried.

WHAT YOU CAN DO AT HOME

If the condition is not severe, keeping the area clean and exposed to air and sunlight may be enough to cure it. Soak the nail and its surrounding skin in hot water, or a brew of goldenseal or echinacea, several times a day, then dry it thoroughly.

Vitamin E oil, apple-cider vinegar, or goldenseal tincture applied directly to the area several times a day may clear up an infection, as may tea-tree oil, or powdered sulphur mixed in olive oil. A lemon or comfrey poultice may be applied once a day for a week (or as long as needed).

Increase vitamins A, C, E, B-complex, trace minerals, and protein in the diet.

INGROWN TOENAILS

If a toenail is cut unevenly, or so short that the underlying skin is exposed, tissue may grow around it and become infected. This can be treated by soaking the toe in a warm brew of goldenseal or calendula, or warm salt water, and gently removing the sloughing skin. A small piece of cotton soaked in castor oil or olive oil mixed with the calendula tincture can be inserted under the nail edge to keep it growing in the right direction, away from the skin. Sandals or shoes with cut-out toes should be worn to keep pressure away from the toe. If the ingrown nail does not heal, a doctor may remove the toenail (though they often grow back ingrown), or remove the whole nailbed and recommend an artificial nail.

FLU (Influenza)

Flu is a common name applied to a wide variety of viral illnesses (more intense than the common cold) whose symptoms include headache, fever, runny nose, sore throat, cough, muscle aches, and sometimes vomiting, diarrhea, and a general feeling of being miserable. These usually last only a few days.

If the symptoms are very intense, however—violent vomiting or diarrhea, extreme pain in the head or spine, an alarming-looking rash or hemorrhaging under the skin—a doctor should be consulted immediately.

WHAT A PHYSICIAN MAY DO

Since flus are usually virus-related, antibiotics will not affect them, although some doctors will prescribe them "to cover all the bases" anyway. If vomiting and diarrhea, fever or respiratory problems are severe, the doctor may want to hospitalize the child (see appropriate sections). New flu vaccines are developed periodically and recommended by some doctors; since there are so many strains of flu around it is unlikely that all of them could be covered in a shot. Flu vaccines have been known to cause many serious side effects, including neurological damage. People often report a decline in their general state of health after receiving flu shots.

WHAT YOU CAN DO AT HOME

PRACTICAL MEASURES. The child should rest in bed and be given lots to drink. Juices, lemon-water, and herb teas are soothing. Warm applications to aching parts (head, chest, back, arms, legs) may soothe the pain.

NUTRITION. The diet should be mostly liquids, especially if digestion is upset. Nutrients that help strengthen the body against infection are vitamins A, C, E, zinc, and pantothenic acid.

HERB TEAS. Rose hips, chamomile, echinacea, peppermint, lemon balm, lemongrass, ginger.

HOMEOPATHIC REMEDIES. (See also COLDS, DIARRHEA, NAUSEA AND VOMITING.)

Arsenicum album. Child is anxious and exhausted, with burning pains relieved by heat; worse after midnight; dislikes the idea or sight or smell of food; thirsty but wants drinks in sips. (Also a good remedy for food poisoning.)

Bryonia. Pain in the abdomen, painful cough; child is grumpy, miserable, very thirsty, with dry mouth and lips; feels worse having to move or being bothered.

China (Cinchona). Fever and chill; gas and watery diarrhea or vomiting that brings on weakness; bursting headache; dizziness; child is distant or irritable.

Eupatorium perfoliatum. Deep aching in bones and eyeballs; ache and heaviness in head; child is chilly, thirsty, feels "wiped out."

Gelsemium. Symptoms come on gradually; headache in back of head; general aching; chills up the back; child is very droopy and lethargic.

Nux vomica. Severe cold symptoms or nausea; child may feel the urge to vomit, but nothing comes up; irritable, sensitive to noise, smells, and being bothered; feels cold, even when covered up.

Phosphorus. Child may be cheerful despite very high fever; colds go into chest; loss of voice; thirst for ice-cold drinks, then the liquid may cause nausea when it warms in the stomach; better from sleep and rubbing.

ACUPRESSURE AND MASSAGE.

LI 11: A tender point at the thumb side end of the elbow-crease when the arm is bent.

ST 36: A tender point next to the outer side of the big bump at the top of the shin.

SP 6: A tender point three of the child's finger-breadths above the inner anklebone.

ST 12: A "gnawed" feeling indentation behind the upper middle of the collarbone.

GV 14: The point at the tip of the big bump in the spine where the neck and upper back meet.

FOREIGN OBJECTS

Small children who like to experiment may, on occasion, push foreign objects into almost any body opening, and find they can't get them out again. This is usually a fairly benign (though often tricky) problem, but it can be an emergency. If an object is lodged in a child's throat or windpipe and is causing choking, suffocation, or unconsciousness, emergency help should be obtained immediately. A foreign object in the eye (see EYE CONDITIONS), in a deep cut, or causing pain or bleeding should also be treated as an emergency.

OBJECTS IN THE RESPIRATORY TRACT

If a child suddenly gasps for breath or is choking, a foreign object may be stuck in her upper air passages. If the object is soft, like a piece of cloth or burst balloon, you can sometimes hook it out with your finger. If you can't, turn the child upside down and give a firm slap between her shoulder blades. If it is still not dislodged, try again. If the child is too big to be turned upside down, use the Heimlich maneuver: stand behind her, place your clasped hands between navel and rib cage (make sure you are not on the ribs), and deliver a quick upward thrust. If the child is very small, or lying down, place the flats of your fingertips between navel and ribcage, and give a gentle but quick thrust headward. You may need to make several attempts; if you are not immediately successful, do *not* stop trying to dislodge the object—but, while doing so, call an emergency squad or rush the child to help. (See section on CHOKING under Emergencies in Part Two.)

A child with a smaller object (such as a bead, pebble, flake of cereal, or popcorn kernel) stuck in his air passages may sometimes be coughing or wheezing but still be able to breathe. Try to get it out by turning him upside down and slapping his back, or use the Heimlich maneuver as described above. If this doesn't work, get professional help right away. Tiny objects can cause big problems if drawn deeper into the lungs.

OBJECTS IN THE DIGESTIVE TRACT

Toddlers, and quite a number of older children, seem unable to resist putting things into their mouths, and often swallow them. Fortunately, most small objects can pass through the digestive tract from mouth to anus without incident. Even tacks and pins have a good chance of passing through without doing much more damage than a scratch in the bottom; during the peristaltic motion that moves material through the intestines, most objects bounce off the folds in the muscular wall and move along. There are places, however, in which an object may become stuck. If an object larger than a nickel, or any sharp object, has been swallowed, it is important to have a doctor's help in monitoring its passage—and, if necessary, getting it out surgically. If a child swallows anything containing chemicals (such as a small button battery), call a doctor.

Chewing slippery-elm tablets or drinking aloe vera gel may help in passing inert swallowed objects.

OBJECTS IN THE NOSE

If some small object like a bean, bead, raisin, or flower bud, has been pushed up a nostril, try the following method of removing it. Hold the unplugged nostril shut and, making a seal with your mouth, blow air into the child's open mouth. Since there is nowhere else for it to go, the air will push through the plugged-up nostril, and often the intruding object pops right out.

Sometimes bad breath or an unexplained runny nose (perhaps with foul-smelling yellow-green discharge or blood in it) means that—unknown to you—the child's nostril has harbored a stranger for several days. If you cannot easily remove the object, a doctor can usually do so with forceps.

OBJECTS IN THE EARS

"Never stick anything smaller than your elbow into your ear" is advice not often followed by small children. It's easy and fun to stuff little things into the ear hole, but much harder to get them out. Unless the object is easily grasped and pulled free, attempts to get it out can damage the sensitive skin of the canal, or even the eardrum and important structures behind it. Never use tweezers or a sharp instrument to try to pry it out; you might push it even farther in.

Check for a foreign object if the child is having trouble hearing, has unusual ear discharge, shakes his head, pulls at an ear, or complains of ear pain without seeming to be sick. If you can't see anything (try a penlight, or an otoscope if you have one), or if you see something but can't get it out with your fingers, call on an expert for help.

OBJECTS IN THE VAGINA OR PENIS

From the time they are very young, children are aware of their genitals as especially sensitive areas, and are likely to experiment with them. Small objects may be pushed inside the openings, eventually causing itching, pain, a bad smell, discharge, or infection. Sometimes in response to the family's attitude toward the genitals, or sometimes from the child's own sense of privacy, the child may not tell you that there is something in there—even if he or she knows there is—and may resist examination. A relaxed cheerful approach will make things easier: tell him or her there's nothing shameful or spooky about it, but any object put where it doesn't belong has to come out, or he or she might not feel well.

FISHHOOKS

Getting a fishhook lodged in the skin is a fairly common injury and can be scary. If the hook is in or near the eye, go for professional help immediately. If it's in a less delicate spot—an earlobe or finger, for instance—the best way to remove it is to snip off the barb with wire-cutters or strong clippers, or thoroughly flatten it with pliers, and slip the hook out backwards. Once this is done, squeeze the wound to make it bleed, since bleeding will help carry dirt out of the wound. Afterwards, clean it thoroughly with soap and water. (For other remedies, see PUNCTURE WOUNDS.)

FRACTURES

Children lead active lives—they jump from swings, topple off skateboards, fall out of trees—and may turn up with the occasional broken bone. These injuries need attention, but usually heal fairly quickly unless the injury is complicated. Because children are growing, their bones are more likely than adults' bones to splinter ("greenstick" fracture) than to receive clean breaks. Also, growing bones have cartilage growth-plates near the joints; if a fracture occurs in the area of a growth-plate, deformity or growth impairment may result unless the injury receives special care. If a child's bones seem to break very easily from what seems to be a minor trauma, consult a physician.

If a child has suffered a hard fall or blow and you think it is possible that a bone has been broken, check for the following symptoms, and if any are found, get medical help right away. Is the limb numb, cold, turning blue? Is the limb crooked? Is the child unable to use or bear weight with the injured limb? Is she pale, sweaty, dizzy, or thirsty? (These are signs of shock. See the shock section in Part Two, and call 911 for help.) When an injured limb looks swollen and bruised, the child complains of pain and refuses to use the limb, or if the injury is near a joint, or there is a great deal of swelling and tenderness that is not much improved over the next forty-eight hours, a fracture should be suspected and a doctor consulted.

WHAT A PHYSICIAN MAY DO

An X ray will usually be taken to see if there is a fracture and, if so, its exact location, type, and extent. It can take several days for the changes that indicate a fracture to show up on X ray; hairline fractures may not show up at all.

The doctor will set (properly align) the ends of the broken bone if necessary. If the limb is crooked and very painful, a general anesthetic may be given to reduce fear, pain, and interfering motion. If the fracture is in the region of a joint, you should be referred to an orthopedic surgeon, and pins may be inserted. A cast or splint may be put on, according to the type of break, and the child will be kept in the hospital if the doctor thinks that observation or surgery may be needed. Sometimes traction is required to keep the bone ends in position for proper healing and to keep them from overlapping or being drawn out of place by swelling or muscle contraction.

Because the procedures for treating a serious fracture are often uncomfortable and frightening, you should find out in detail from the doctor what to expect so you can explain it to your child in a way he can understand. Stay with the child as much as you can. (You might bring a foam-rubber pad and sleeping bag and stay in the hospital room.) If an anesthetic is used, tell your child ahead of time how he might feel afterwards, and what procedures the doctor might apply—such as a splint, cast, or traction—so the child's pain and restriction are not compounded by fear.

If the child has to be immobilized a long time, make sure he has lots of company and keep him engaged and amused as much as possible so he doesn't panic. Sometimes it takes a long time for a serious injury to heal, and it is expecting too much of a child (or an adult) who is accustomed to moving freely and being active to just "get used to it."

WHAT YOU CAN DO AT HOME

Home care measures alone are *not* sufficient for treating a fracture. If you suspect one, call a doctor within the first few days.

PRACTICAL MEASURES. The limb should be placed in the most comfortable position, and the child should rest. If the child is able to move, and the limb is not distorted or bleeding, put ice packs on the hurt areas as soon as possible, to decrease inflammation and swelling. A splint can be made to keep the hurt limb still and keep the joints above and below the injury from moving. Rolled newspaper or cardboard may work as splints, wrapped securely with a bandage; or the injured leg may be splinted against the good one, or a broken arm bound to the child's side. Do not wrap splints too tightly, since the area will be swelling. Binding a poultice of comfrey leaves on the injured part every day for several weeks can help.

NUTRITION. Give extra vitamin C, calcium, magnesium, phosphorus, trace minerals, and B-complex to help the surrounding tissues heal. Make sure the child has adequate vitamin D and plenty of moderate sunlight. Pay special attention to the child's nutrition, making sure he gets plenty of protein and fresh fruit and vegetables. Watch for problems in digestion and assimilation. Chewing on comfrey leaves or drinking comfrey tea can help fractures heal.

HOMEOPATHIC REMEDIES. "Rescue Remedy," a combination of Bach Flower Remedies used in emergencies, can be given right after the injury. *Arnica* should be given at first to help bruised tissues and ease pain and shock; later, *Symphytum* is useful to help the bones rejoin and heal.

ACUPRESSURE AND MASSAGE.
> BL 11: The points in the muscles two of the child's thumb-widths to the sides of the vertebra below the bony bump at the base of the neck.
> LI 4: The point at the end of the crease between the thumb and index finger.
> KI 3: The tender point just behind the upper rear aspect of the inner anklebone.

FUNGUS INFECTIONS

When resistance to infection is down, the skin can be susceptible to the growth of fungus, which thrives in warm, damp, sweaty areas.

Ringworm is the most common fungus condition in children, appearing on the skin and hairy areas. (See also HAIR AND SCALP.) It isn't really a worm; the fungus causes small red bumps to form in a ring that spreads outward as the center heals. Ringworm can itch very badly, but doesn't always.

Athlete's foot is usually seen between the toes, as cracked, whitish, itchy skin. It can spread to the tops of the feet or the nails, but doesn't very often.

"Jock itch" consists of patches of itchy redness that start in the crotch and spread several inches down the thighs. It is usually seen in older, athletic boys.

WHAT A PHYSICIAN MAY DO

A doctor will likely recommend salicylic acid preparations or un
decylenic acid medications available in drugstores (e.g., Tinactin
for ringworm, Desenex for athlete's foot). Some doctors prescribe
the drug griseofulvin to be taken orally; its side effects may be digestive upset, skin rashes, and decrease in white blood cells. Since
a tendency to fungal infection indicates weakened immune function, suppression of eruptions with chemicals is probably not the
best solution.

WHAT YOU CAN DO AT HOME

PRACTICAL MEASURES. Most fungus conditions go away by themselves in time. They are, however, very contagious. Do not let children touch animals or persons with skin eruptions or patchy hair
loss unless you know the condition has a noncontagious cause.
Encourage them not to use other people's brushes and combs
or wear others' hats or shoes.

Keep skin clean and dry. Wear loose clothing to let air circulate; expose the skin to moderate sunlight. Have the child wear
white cotton socks and underwear.

NATURAL APPLICATIONS. Lemon juice, apple-cider vinegar, crushed
garlic, castor oil, or egg white can be dabbed on the spots several
times a day. Strong brews of goldenseal or chaparral, or pastes of
powdered sulphur and olive oil, crushed B-vitamin tablets mixed
with water, or borax in water can be helpful.

NUTRITION. Extra vitamins A, C, B-complex, and zinc help the
skin resist infection. Include acidophilus (in capsules or tablets or
cultured yogurt and kefir) and several tablespoons of sunflower
oil in the daily diet.

HOMEOPATHIC REMEDIES.

> *Graphites.* Oozing cracks between the toes, offensive foot sweat;
> ringworm, with sticky, golden-colored crusts; child may be over-
> weight, and deeply moved by music.
> *Petroleum.* Skin between the toes is red, raw, and cracked; itching
> at night; child may have tendency to motion sickness, heartburn.
> *Rhus toxicodendron.* Tingling, red swelling of toes; itching
> relieved by hot water; humid ringworm, especially on the scalp
> and face; child feels better moving around.

Sepia. Ringworm that turns brown and itches or burns, worse in bends of knees and elbows; may recur each spring; child feels better from exercise.

Sulphur. Skin is dry, red, irritated with itching and burning; worse from warmth and scratching; child may dislike bathing.

GROWTH

Parents sometimes worry that their child is not growing at the proper rate, and wonder whether to take him to a physician for tests and screening. Usually these fears are needless. If your child is mentally alert, has a good appetite and plenty of energy, don't worry too much about the height and weight charts. Children are individuals: not everyone has to be "average" to be normal.

Rarely, certain diseases, nutritional deficiencies, or hormonal imbalances (usually from impaired function of the pituitary or thyroid glands) will make a child grow too slowly or keep him from developing normally. If the child's growth seems strange—for instance, if the head or chest is distorted or any bones seem weak or painful—check with a doctor.

WHAT A PHYSICIAN MAY DO

If the doctor suspects that the child's development is abnormal even with adequate nutrition, she will probably take X rays to check the presence of normal growth-plates in the wrist bones, and assess the age of the bone material. Blood and metabolic tests may also be run to check production of thyroid, pituitary, and sex hormones and to assess the efficiency of and balance between the functions of the endocrine glands. If the tests indicate an endocrine problem, hormone therapy may be recommended. Be cautious: hormone therapy can be harmful and is only justified for extreme problems. Before submitting to any of the above procedures, which are somewhat invasive and expensive, you may prefer to get opinions from several doctors, including those who use homeopathy, cranial manipulations, and acupuncture for such cases.

WHAT YOU CAN DO AT HOME

PRACTICAL MEASURES. Heredity is the main factor in a child's growth pattern and size. Think about the size and growth histories of the child's relatives, especially parents and grandparents. Sometimes tall parents have a few small relatives here and there in their family trees; tall members of the family may be carrying short-person genes and may produce a short child. Many children remain small through adolescence, then suddenly have a growth spurt when puberty arrives—ending up tall, or at least of average size. Get a growth chart and mark your child's progress; growing *consistently* is more important than being some desired size at a certain point in time.

NUTRITION. Children need a well-balanced and varied diet to supply the building blocks for growth. Several ounces of good-quality protein per day (from whole grains, nuts, dairy products, eggs, fish, or meat) is extremely important, as are fresh fruits and vegetables. The less refined and processed food a growing child consumes, the better chance he has of growing and developing well.

Vitamin and mineral supplements should provide balanced B-complex vitamins, vitamins C and E, adequate vitamins A and D (which help the body use minerals for good bone growth), calcium, magnesium, zinc, and vital trace minerals such as manganese, chromium, and selenium.

HOMEOPATHIC REMEDIES. Treatment with constitutional remedies is helpful to children with problems in growth and development. Among those often prescribed (when specifically indicated) are *Baryta carbonica, Calcarea phosphorica, Calcarea carbonica,* and *Phosphorus.* If a child's condition is serious, seek the help of an expert prescriber.

Hair and Scalp

Although the color, texture, and thickness of a person's hair are determined by heredity, the gloss and resilience of a child's hair may reflect her state of nutrition and vitality. Dull hair or hair that breaks easily may mean that the child needs better-quality protein and minerals. Oats, whole grains, seeds, nuts, sprouts, and raw vegetables provide the element silicon, which helps strengthen the nails and hair. Hair can also lack luster if circulation to the scalp is poor. Massage of the scalp, gentle vertebral adjustments, and B vitamins (including niacin) can help.

HAIR LOSS

Hair loss in children can be caused by severe nutritional deficiencies, low thyroid or adrenal function, or vitamin A toxicity, but seems often to be a result of emotional and nervous strain. Attempts should be made to discover any emotional tensions and pressures and help the child deal with them. Massaging the scalp to improve circulation is helpful and may also be relaxing to the child. A tea made of nettle and sage, rubbed, lukewarm, into the scalp after each shampoo can help.

Nutrition is important, especially the B vitamins, biotin, PABA, choline, and inositol, and vitamin E. Onions and oats or other silicon-rich foods are helpful.

Sometimes a child pulls out his own hair as a nervous habit (or sometimes, in too-rough play, a friend might do it for him). Occasionally, hair that has been too tightly braided or pushed back repeatedly with a plastic headband will break off. If hair falls out in patches, but the scalp is normal underneath, it will usually grow back within several months.

RINGWORM

This highly contagious fungus infection is often found on children's scalps. Wearing a hat or using a brush belonging to someone with the infection, or nuzzling a cat that carried it, may be enough to pick up ringworm. A little ring of blisters forms and expands outward as the center heals. The hair in these patches falls out but later grows back. (See FUNGUS INFECTIONS.)

CRADLE CAP (Seborrhea)

Cradle cap is a condition that looks like greasy, scaly, yellowish or brown dandruff, seen on the scalps and eyebrows of some babies and toddlers, especially those whose hair is blond. It comes from oil glands in the skin that do not yet clear themselves properly. It isn't dangerous and will eventually go away, but some people dislike the way it looks. A gentle way to remove it is to apply a little warm olive or rosemary oil to the scaly patches, leave it on for about fifteen minues, and then peel it off with a clean toothbrush or comb. Afterwards, the hair may have to be shampooed more than once to get rid of the "'50's greaser" look. Cradle cap may come back several times, but eventually the oil glands catch on to their job. Some children who have had cradle cap have problems with dandruff later on. Supplements of biotin and vitamin B_6 along with B-complex in moderate doses may clear it up in such cases. Constitutional homeopathic treatment is also helpful.

DANDRUFF

Dandruff can be an oil-gland condition, like cradle cap, or may be a result of allergy, poor digestion, poor nutrition, or emotional stress. Eliminating refined flour, sugar, and processed foods from the diet is often enough to make dandruff go away. Include lots of fresh foods in the diet, especially alfalfa sprouts, carrots, beets, and other raw fruits and vegetables, and give the child extra B-complex vitamins.

Flaking and itchy scalp could be a reaction to an irritating shampoo. Changing to a gentle natural shampoo may help, as may giving the hair extra rinses after washing. After the hair is clean, apple-cider vinegar can be applied to the scalp. Herb teas made of mint and nettle may be used as rinses, rubbed into the scalp, and also taken internally.

It is best not to use dandruff shampoos containing chemicals such as selenium sulfide on children. Sometimes, for extreme cases, a doctor might recommend cortisone cream; since this can upset the child's hormonal balance, and is not adding anything to the child's health—only changing the symptoms—it is better to stick with the safer approaches. (See ALLERGIES, ECZEMA.) Constitutional homeopathy is often helpful.

HEAD (Cranial) CONDITIONS
(see also HEAD INJURIES)

Newborn babies may normally have somewhat misshapen heads, because the bones of the skull have not yet grown together. The fontanels ("soft spots") on the top and back of the head are areas between the growing bones, covered by membranes as strong as canvas; these openings allow the skull to change shape to absorb the pressure the head receives during birth. Around age two, the fontanels close; up to then, the child's brain is growing very rapidly.

Newborns may also have other odd-looking but harmless head conditions resulting from the rigors of being born: *Caput succedaneum* is a swelling and bruising under the scalp. A *cephalohematoma* is a collection of blood under the membranous covering of a portion of the skull. These don't need treatment—they disappear on their own within a couple of months.

Many children, notably those who had difficult births or were delivered using forceps, continue to have misshapen heads or poorly aligned jaws. These conditions may contribute to dental (bite) problems or jaw-joint (TMJ) difficulties. Children with cranial misalignments or distortions sometimes show symptoms of intracranial tension, such as habitual banging of the head against the wall or crib, sleep troubles, headaches, eye or ear disorders, and behavior problems.

Some cranial distortions can be diagnosed and corrected through gentle manipulation by chiropractors, naturopaths, osteopaths, or other physicians who have devoted special study and practice to cranial work. Parents looking for help in this area should be careful to choose a practitioner who is very experienced in the cranial techniques and experienced with children. Since these manipulations are intended to remove conditions that impede the circulation of cerebrospinal fluid and blood to the brain and nerve centers, they are dealing with very important and often delicate areas and can have a potent effect. Although they often bring dramatic relief, they can also be dangerous if there is a serious underlying health condition, or if they are not properly performed.

HEAD INJURIES

A child who has never had a bump on the head is either exceptionally lucky or just not very active. Children are famous for recovering from head injuries quickly and with no lasting ill effects, since the skull is designed to protect the brain from the occasional fall or knock. In very small children the joints between the skull bones are not fully closed, thus the tough, leathery fontanel or "soft spot" on top of the head also acts to absorb shock. Still, a very hard fall or blow on the head, or violent shaking (such as may occur in a car wreck) can bruise the brain and cause a concussion.

Indications of a concussion include: headache, dizziness, giddiness, lethargy, vomiting, unconsciousness (even for a few seconds), trouble with balance, blurry vision, slurred speech, fluid or blood coming out of the nose or ears, pale clammy skin, or dilated pupils. If any of these are evident, check with a doctor.

If there is *any* possibility that the head and spine are injured seriously, or if the child has memory loss, difficulty moving her arms and legs, irregular breathing, convulsion, change of personality, or if the pupils of her eyes appear to be unequal, keep her still and call for emergency help at once.

WHAT A PHYSICIAN MAY DO

The child's general appearance will be observed, and pulse rate and blood pressure taken. The doctor will examine eyes, ears, nose, throat, neck, and nerve responses, as well as checking for injury to other parts of the body, especially the abdomen and limbs. Sometimes X rays are taken of the head or neck, depending on the nature of the injury or accident. Skull X rays rarely give useful information until an injury is several days old, so they should probably not be taken at first unless the doctor has reason to suspect a specific type of fracture.

Most doctors do not prescribe medications with head injuries because it is important not to obscure any concussion symptoms that might develop in the hours or days following the injury. If the injury is very serious, hospitalization and surgery may be recommended. Otherwise, home care is prescribed.

WHAT YOU CAN DO AT HOME

PRACTICAL MEASURES. If it seems to be an uncomplicated bump, put ice in a towel and hold it on the hurt place to reduce swelling. (For other natural remedies, see BRUISES.) Some minor injuries create huge purple goose-eggs, but many serious injuries hardly show externally. If a little child is crying with pain or outrage, it is usually a sign that the injury isn't too bad.

Have the child lie down and observe him: watch for shock, make sure the pupils are of equal size. He may be drowsy after a head bump, and may even throw up once or twice, but watch for disorientation or other concussion symptoms. A nap is a good remedy; let him sleep but check him every few minutes to be sure he is breathing normally and isn't clammy or cold. Wake him gently every half hour or so to check his pupil size, then let him go back to sleep if he wants to.

HOMEOPATHIC REMEDIES. *Arnica* is good first aid for both shock and bruising. See an experienced homeopath for extended effects of head injuries. Cranial and spinal manipulations from gentle, experienced chiropractors, craniosacral therapists, and osteopaths may also help recovery.

HEADACHES

Some children never have headaches, and some get them only along with a cold or flu, but certain children (and adults) seem inclined to have them frequently for many different resons. There are many causes of headaches. Following is a list of some the most common.

MUSCLE TENSION
When the muscles that connect the neck and shoulders to the back and sides of the head become tight, a headache may be the result. Neck and shoulder muscle tension is often caused by emotional pressure, but may also come from postures that prevent relaxation, such as sitting bent forward at a desk for long periods, or reading in bed without having the neck and shoulders propped up. Tension may also have its source in long-term exposure to irritating noise, extremes of heat and cold, or from a lack of certain nutrients, particularly calcium and magnesium. Misalignments of the spinal vertebrae, allergies and hay fever, eyestrain, colds, sore throats, and ear infections are also contributors.

SPECIFIC NATURAL MEASURES. Contracting and relaxing the tense muscles, massage, and recreational exercise can help relax tense muscles. Give whole grains, fresh fruits and vegetables, plenty of fluids, extra B-vitamins, calcium, and magnesium. Chamomile tea may be relaxing. (See also general remedies at end of chapter.)

LOW BLOOD SUGAR (Hypoglycemia)

This is a likely suspect if a child wakes up most mornings with a headache or gets headaches from skipping meals. Poor nutrition is often responsible for low blood sugar. Most people who eat too much sugar have hypoglycemic episodes because concentrated sweets cause the level of sugar in the blood to rise dramatically, then, as the body summons its resources to combat this stressful situation, it falls just as dramatically.

SPECIFIC NATURAL MEASURES. If your child has a tendency toward hypoglycemia, it is best kept under control by giving her small, frequent meals. If going for even a short time without food causes fatigue, irritability, or headache, have the child carry snacks of complex carbohydrates and protein, whole-grain crackers, nuts, or cheese everywhere she goes. These foods release fuel steadily to the child's system so there is no dramatic fluctuation in glucose, as there may be when sugar or concentrated sweets are eaten. B-complex vitamins and chromium (found in brewer's yeast, nuts, blackstrap molasses, meat, and seafood) are helpful. (See also general remedies at end of chapter.)

DIGESTIVE DIFFICULTIES

Headaches, especially in the sides of the head and forehead, can accompany a stomach upset, gas, or constipation. Attention to nutrition and eating habits will be helpful. (See appropriate sections, as well as general remedies at end of this chapter.)

INFECTION AND ILLNESS

Headaches caused by dehydration or changes in the blood's chemical balance due to fever, vomiting, or diarrhea often accompany children's illnesses. Sometimes inflammations in the ears, nose, tonsils and adenoids, jaw, or sinuses will refer pain to the head and face; in children under six the sinuses are not well developed, so such infections are rare. (For treatment, see appropriate sections; also general remedies at end of this chapter.)

If a sick child has a severe headache, stiff neck with difficulty touching his chin to his chest, seems very irritable or lethargic, has a high fever, and shows a rash or pinpoint bleeding under the skin, a doctor should be seen immediately. (See MENINGITIS.)

EYESTRAIN

In eyestrain, the pain is usually felt in the forehead and in or behind the eyes, and is made worse by a concentrated use of the eyes, such as reading or watching television for long periods of time. Some children have eyestrain headaches every day after school. (School can induce headaches for other reasons, too: emotional pressures, desks or chairs that cause bad posture, fluorescent lighting, lack of fresh air and exercise.) Computer screens, video games, and television are common sources of eyestrain. Some children become absorbed in a favorite activity—reading, writing, drawing, stamp collecting, embroidery, model-making— for hours at a time, oblivious to the need for good lighting or the occasional need to rest their eyes. Such concentration—a thing many grown-ups wish they could muster—must not be discouraged, but parents should make an effort to see that the child has a good, well-lit environment for his work, and has opportunities for outdoor play, natural light, and fresh air.

SPECIFIC NATURAL MEASURES. Massaging the neck and temples may give some relief in cases of eyestrain. Also try rubbing or applying fingertip pressure to tender spots below the base of the skull (behind the ear), to the points at both corners of the eyes, and to the spot just below the ridge of bone at the inner aspect of each eyebrow.

If eyestrain headaches continue, the child should be examined by an ophthalmologist to find out if glasses, a change in lenses, or eye exercises are needed. If the ophthalmologist does not think the headaches come from the eyes, you may be referred to another physician to screen for other causes. (See also general remedies at end of chapter.)

EXPOSURE TO TOXINS

Headaches can come from poisons, medicines, or environmental toxins. Some people get frequent headaches from breathing city air laden with fumes, lead, and carbon monoxide from factories and car exhaust. It is not unknown for industries and individuals to indiscriminately and illegally (and inexpensively) dispose of dangerous poisons by dumping them in woodlands or vacant lots;

children may play there and be exposed to them. Children's headaches could alert you to such problems—but other effects of these chemicals are much worse than headaches.

Children may also have headaches as side effects of medications, or from chewing on objects made of some kinds of plastic or containing certain paints or glues. Serious headaches may also come from sniffing household chemicals, varnish, typist's correction fluid, or pesticides.

SPECIFIC NATURAL MEASURES. MGive a child extra vitamins C, E, and B-complex to help the body fend off toxins. Make sure he drinks lots of liquids, has plenty of exercise, rest, and fresh air. (See also general remedies at end of chapter.)

MIGRAINE

Migraines are very painful headaches, often felt on only one side of the head. The child may first see colored spots or zigzags of light, or have blurry vision, followed by a terrible throbbing headache that can be accompanied by nausea, vomiting, weakness, chills, or sweating. Migraines are different from other headaches in that they seem to come from an overreaction of blood vessels in the scalp and brain: some vessels constrict (become narrow), then some dilate (widen) and are stretched with extra blood; some may constrict again. This can create severe pain and may alter various functions of the brain tissue, causing the other symptoms.

Many children who regularly get these devastating headaches have what is known as the "migraine personality." High-strung and bright, they expect a lot of themselves, and often come down with a migraine when—after successfully passing through a time of stress—they have the opportunity to relax.

There is often a period of unjustified irritability or elation before the headache comes on. Sometimes the first sign of a migraine is an aversion to food—even though eating a snack before it's too late may lessen or avert the headache by raising the blood-sugar level.

Migraines may occur every week, or once a month, or only one or two may occur in a lifetime. They may be hereditary, and in most cases seem to have a connection with food allergy. Migraine sufferers may be allergic to many different things at once. Foods such as wheat, chocolate, cheese, nuts, bananas, grapes, citrus fruits, dried apricots, cola drinks, black tea, and wine are often connected to migraine—but any substance could do it, depending on the sensitivities of the individual child. Chemicals and additives such as nitrates and nitrites, MSG, sulfites, and artificial sweeteners can trigger migraine. During times of stress, the liver may not be able to efficiently break down the substances that trigger migraine, to clear them from the bloodstream. This may be why migraines often show up in girls near the age of puberty when hormones begin to make dramatic shifts.

Some people have found that migraines can be staved off by home remedies, if the headache is caught in time. Unfortunately, the preheadache period often includes a mood of apathy or irascibility; the child may need to be coerced into admitting that a headache is coming and that something needs to be done about it.

FIRST AID FOR MIGRAINE

Have the child keep her feet in a tub of very warm water, while someone holds an ice pack on the back of her neck.

Have the child take a brisk walk or engage in ten or fifteen minutes of vigorous exercise. This is sometimes useful to ward off the blood-vessel reaction, but should be done at the first sign of an oncoming headache. The child will probably not feel like exercising once the headache is under way.

Give a teaspoonful of honey; it contains natural sugars and trace minerals and sometimes is enough to thwart an early migraine.

Give 100 mg of niacin to expand constricting blood vessels; it may also cause flushing of the skin.

Give sips of strong black coffee or espresso. This is only for first aid: coffee is *not* a healthy drink for children, but an exception can be made if a migraine is coming on. Caffeine affects the blood-vessel spasms that bring on symptoms; caffeine is an active ingredient in drugs often prescribed by doctors to treat migraine. *(Note: If you plan to use homeopathic remedies, do not use coffee; it will interfere with them.)*

HERB TEAS. Basil, fennel, hops, lavender, nettle, peppermint, shepherd's purse, speedwell, yerba maté. (See also general remedies at end of chapter.)

Migraine is a deep disorder and needs more than symptomatic treatment. Constitutional homeopathy, cranial and spinal manipulations, acupuncture and Chinese herbal therapy, and specific nutritional programs have been beneficial to children who suffer from migraine. Consult experienced practitioners for these.

OTHER CAUSES. Other causes of headaches include: anemia, crying, cranial or jaw misalignments (TMJ problems), and head injuries. Aneurysms and tumors in the nervous system can also cause headaches but are very rare. If a child with headaches experiences behavior changes, dizziness, one-sided muscle weakness, difficulties in speaking or seeing, ear noises, vomiting or unconsciousness, see a doctor immediately.

WHAT A PHYSICIAN MAY DO

Most doctors will examine the child, looking for signs of infection, muscle tension, poisoning, or eyestrain; blood tests and urine tests may be done to check for infection, anemia, allergy, or metabolic problems. Some recommend pain medications such as aspirin and acetaminophen, or prescribe more potent pain killers. Although aspirin is a very common drug, easily available, and almost the universal prescription for headaches, it can also have dangerous effects and should not be given to children. Acetaminophen, another common headache medicine, has also been known to cause some side effects when it is ingested, again, so it should be avoided. For severe headaches or migraine, a doctor may prescribe caffeine-ergot preparations that affect the dilation and constriction of blood vessels. Some give codeine, an addictive narcotic. Some give inderal, a drug with many side effects, usually prescribed for blood-pressure abnormalities. Make the effort to find natural remedies and therapies that work for your child; they are much safer.

WHAT YOU CAN DO AT HOME

PRACTICAL MEASURES. Make sure the child has plenty of fresh air and exercise, a chance to relax and have fun every day. Give neck- and head-rubs and back massage.

NUTRITION. Make sure the diet is free of refined foods and chemical additives. A balanced vitamin and mineral supplement should be given; include extra vitamins C, B-complex, calcium, and magnesium.

HERB TEAS. Peppermint, chamomile, lemon juice, basil, thyme, ginger, fennel, nettle, rose hips.

HOMEOPATHIC REMEDIES.

Aconitum napellus. Sudden, violent, bursting headache, especially in the forehead, or like a band around the head; child feels frightened, panicky; thirsty; worse at night.

Arnica montana. Headache from a head injury or fall; head feels bruised inside; child may not want to be touched.

Belladonna. Pounding head pain, throbbing pulse, dilated eyes that are sensitive to light; child is often feverish with a flushed face, can be delirious.

Bryonia. Steady ache, which may settle over the left eye; nausea; can come on after a stressful day or from eyestrain; any motion makes the pain worse.

Calcarea phosphorica. Sweaty head; roots of the hair seem to hurt; worse from jarring, wearing a hat, weather changes; child is anemic, dissatisfied, loves junk food.

Gelsemium. Ache in neck and back of head spreads to forehead, settles over eye or temple; like a band around the head; tender scalp; heavy eyelids; vision disturbed; worse from light and noise; child very drowsy; better after urinating.

Ignatia. Pain like a nail in the head or cramping in face or nose; worse from stooping, worse from smelling tobacco smoke; better after eating; emotional upsets, anger, grief.

Iris versicolor. Blurry vision, burning tongue and throat; nausea, salivation, vomiting; pain often right-sided; child feels better moving around in open air.

Kali bichromium. Intense pain in very small spots: forehead, sinus area, face; bones and scalp feel sore; vertigo on standing up; worse from motion; better in open air.

Natrum muriaticum. Frequent headaches from eyestrain, mental exertion, long trips, movie-going. If the child needs this remedy, it should be given constitutionally, not in the midst of a headache. If a headache is very bad, give *Bryonia* or *Ignatia* (if either fits), and give *Natrum muriaticum* later, for the chronic condition.

Nux vomica. Whole head aches; after overeating, indigestion, or missing sleep; child is irritable; worse in morning; better in evening, from warmth, or from lying down.

Sanguinaria. Splitting, throbbing pain from back of head into right eye; worse from sun; better in dark, after vomiting, or from hard pressure on head and neck.

Silicea. Ache starts at back of neck, comes up over head to eyes; worse from pressure, from missing meals; head feels cold and child wants it covered; child may find school stressful, even if doing well.

Spigelia. Pain deep in eyes, forehead, temples; pulsating, often left-sided; stiff neck and shoulders; worse from warmth and motion; better from cold applications.

ACUPRESSURE AND MASSAGE.

LU 7: The tender point on the undersurface of the thumb-side forearm bone, two of the child's thumb-widths above the palm-size wrist-crease.

LI 4: The point at the end of the crease between the thumb and index finger.

· Massage tender points in the muscles where the base of the skull joins the neck.

· Massage the bump on the lower knuckle of the thumb on the index finger side.

HEARING PROBLEMS
(see also EAR CONDITIONS)

Hearing problems in children may be temporary or permanent, depending on the cause. Total deafness in children is not common, but degrees of deafness (often undetected) occur frequently for many reasons. There are two types of deafness: sensorineural, due to damage to the eighth cranial nerve (also called the auditory or acoustic nerve) or to structures in the inner ear; and conductive, caused by damage or obstruction in the ear canal and middle ear.

Sensorineural deafness may be the result of an extremely loud noise, such as an explosion, or repeated exposure to loud sounds (e.g., living near a noisy factory, playing in a rock band, listening to blasting headphones). The acoustic nerve may also be damaged by a violent blow to the ear or a severe concussion. Exposure to certain poisons can also lead to nerve deafness: environmental toxins such as arsenic and mercury, medications such as quinine, streptomycin and similar antibiotics—even too much aspirin—can cause deafness or noises in the ears; drinking a lot of alcohol may also permanently affect the hearing nerves. Very high fevers, and complications from diseases such as meningitis, strep infections, syphilis, diphtheria, leukemia, and very severe cases of measles, mumps, or chicken pox can cause nerve deafness. Babies are often born deaf if their mothers had German measles (rubella) during the first three months of pregnancy, or were given shots for rubella not knowing they were pregnant. (Some women contract rubella while pregnant, expecting to be immune because of a previous vaccination that has "worn off.")

Conductive hearing loss can be caused by blocking of the ear canal by too much wax or a foreign object. During a head cold, congestion and swelling of membranes may block the eustachian tubes, changing the pressure inside the ear, or the middle ear may fill with fluid or pus due to an ear infection and temporarily interfere with the transmission of sound. Chronic infection can cause scarring that will permanently impair hearing. Growths or boils in the ear can also block passage of sound.

A baby who does not show the startle reflex (jerking or crying when a sudden loud noise occurs nearby) or, after the age of nine months, does not turn his head toward a prominent unexpected sound, may have hearing problems. If a child has not learned to talk by the age of two, or does not speak in sentences, by around age three, does not express feelings and wants verbally, seems not to hear what is said to him, talks very loudly (even in a normal, unexcited mood), or frequently mishears words that are spoken clearly (for example, confuses the sounds *p* and *b*), it would be wise to have his hearing tested.

WHAT A PHYSICIAN MAY DO

A doctor will examine the child and look in the ears for signs of infection, foreign bodies, or blockage. A tuning-fork test may be performed to determine whether hearing loss is due to problems with conduction or sense perception; an audiometer may be used to estimate the degree of nerve deafness. Ear specialists (otologists) use special diagnostic equipment to find particular points of damage, tumors, or obstructions that might be interfering with nerve function. Based on the history of your child's hearing problem and an examination, an otologist will consider whether surgery is likely to correct the problem. Hearing aids, which do not cure deafness but can augment hearing in a child who is partially deaf, are sometimes prescribed. Speech and hearing clinics may provide different sorts of therapy, such as lipreading and sign language, to give a child with limited hearing other skills for communicating.

WHAT YOU CAN DO AT HOME

PRACTICAL MEASURES. If hearing loss comes on suddenly, check the ear canals for foreign objects (some children like to put things into any body opening, just "because it's there"). Try to remove only those objects that are easily grasped; pull out only, do not push in. Be gentle: remember that the eardrum is not far away, and the ear canal is very sensitive. If the object doesn't come out easily, get help from an expert.

If the ear canal is full of wax, rather than gouging at it with a swab (which may just jam it farther in), have the child sit in a hot bath a while to liquefy the wax, then wipe it out of the outer hole with a washcloth; massaging the fleshy part of the ear, and the points in front and behind, helps loosen wax. Drugstores sell small ear-irrigation kits that doctors may recommend for home use if earwax tends to become impacted. These should be used (if at all) only in ears that are totally free of infection, using tepid water mixed with antiseptic drops. Never put anything very cold or hot in the ear, as this can cause dizziness and nausea.

Do not let children put their ears close to stereo speakers, shoot off cap guns near their ears, or be close to extremely loud noises for any length of time.

NUTRITION. General good nutrition to prevent infection and allergy can help prevent hearing loss. Vitamins C and A, raw garlic and onions, and the herb summer savory have been of use especially in cases for which no particular cause of hearing problems has been found.

HOMEOPATHIC REMEDIES. A constitutional remedy from an experienced prescriber may improve hearing.

ACUPRESSURE AND MASSAGE. Treatment with acupuncture and Chinese herbs from an experienced practitioner may help some cases of hearing loss.

· Rub the areas in front of and behind the ear where it attaches to the head.
· Massage the neck and upper back muscles, especially tender areas.
  KI 1: A point on the sole between the pads of the ball of the foot.
  KI 3: The tender point just behind the upper rear aspect of the inner anklebone.

HEPATITIS

Hepatitis is an illness in which the liver is inflamed. In children the disease may be mild or severe and is often related to a virus that is spread through poor sanitation or sewage-contaminated water, or from person to person. The liver may also become inflamed after exposure to certain toxins or drugs; this sort of hepatitis is not infectious.

The first symptoms may seem like the flu—nausea at the sight of food, loss of appetite, low-grade fever (102 degrees F. or so), muscle aches, headache, and tiredness. The liver (located in the abdomen, just under the right side of the rib cage) may feel heavy or be tender when pressed. Sometimes the urine becomes dark and the bowel movements light-colored. Jaundice, which causes the skin and eyewhites to look yellow, may appear, but often does not show up until the child has been ill for a week or more. After about two weeks, it is unlikely that the child will pass the infection on to anyone else, but relapses of the symptoms can occur during the next few months, and the child is likely to feel very tired.

Children rarely catch hepatitis, because a healthy liver seldom lets the disease take hold; most children's livers are fairly clean, not having been exposed to as many poisons and unhealthy living habits as have those of many adults. However, an infant may contract hepatitis from an unhealthy mother; or a child who consumes impure water or food (often a concern when traveling) may catch the disease.

WHAT A PHYSICIAN MAY DO

There are blood tests for detecting hepatitis, but they are not always accurate. If the child has hepatitis symptoms but the blood test is negative, the doctor may try to determine whether other causes, such as clogged bile ducts, mononucleosis, poisoning, or drugs, are contributing.

The only beneficial treatment prescribed for hepatitis by conventional doctors consists of rest, adequate nourishment, and time. Avoiding the use of contaminated or suspicious water—for drinking, swimming, or as a source of seafood—can help protect children (and adults) against contracting hepatitis. Family members and anyone exposed or expecting to be exposed to hepatitis may be given gamma globulin shots to keep their immunity high.

Alternative medical approaches such as homeopathy, acupuncture, and Chinese herbal therapy are often successful in aiding recovery from hepatitis. Consult an experienced practitioner.

WHAT YOU CAN DO AT HOME

NUTRITION. Hepatitis is too serious an illness to be treated without a physician's monitoring, but the liver may be cleansed and strengthened by following a diet that consists mostly of fruits and vegetables and their juices, especially oranges, grapefruits, lemons, tomatoes, and sauerkraut. Also, small amounts of easily digestible, good-quality protein, such as eggs or lean chicken or fish, and several tablespoonfuls of cold-pressed oils (such as sesame, sunflower, or wheat-germ oil) should be given.

Vitamin C—100 mg or more per hour—can help the body overcome the viral infection. A basic multimineral-multivitamin supplement should be given to help raise the body's resistance, but vitamin A should not be oversupplied (5,000 IU per day is enough), as the liver is sensitive to it.

HERB TEAS. Dandelion, echinacea, peppermint, lemon balm.

HOMEOPATHIC REMEDIES. If a child is very ill, see a homeopathic physician.

ACUPRESSURE AND MASSAGE.
LV 3: A tender point midway between the first and second metatarsal bones.

LV 14: A tender point on the front of the rib cage, midway between the nipple and the lower ribs.

ST 36: A tender point next to the outer side of the big bump at the top of the shin.

SP 6: A tender point three of the child's finger-breadths above the inner anklebone.

· Massage along the spine from mid- to lower back.

HICCUPS

Hiccups happen when the diaphragm (the dome-shaped muscular partition that divides the chest from the abdomen) goes into sudden spasmodic contraction and causes a sharp intake of breath. The opening at the top of the larynx snaps shut, making the famous sound.

The cause of a case of hiccups can't always be tracked down. Small babies seem to have frequent bouts of them without being bothered. Hiccups may show up when a child is excited, anxious, or nervous (emotional tension is often held in the diaphragm), after eating spicy food, eating or drinking too quickly (especially carbonated beverages or very hot drinks), or from exercise right after a meal. They may accompany other digestive or respiratory disturbances.

A hiccup attack can last a few minutes to several hours, or even days. Some hiccups hurt; some are fun; some are a nuisance. If they last more than a day and don't respond to any home cures, it might be helpful to check with a physician. (Very rarely, prolonged hiccups come from infections, or even tumors.)

Human beings breathe in to take in oxygen, and breathe out to get rid of carbon dioxide (CO_2, a by-product of metabolism). It seems that hiccups are accentuated when the CO_2 in the blood is low. Ways of inhibiting hiccups by raising the child's CO_2 level, or by relieving pressure on the phrenic nerve, include:

· Have the child hold her breath as long as she can; repeat till hiccups are gone.
· Have her breathe in and out inside a paper bag (*not* a plastic one).
· Have her drink a big glass of water without stopping, while her ears are plugged.

- Give her a glass of water and have her bend her neck, in order to place her mouth on the far lip of the glass, and drink it "backwards."

  Other remedies that often work:
- Give the child fresh orange juice, dried sweetened coconut, or a teaspoonful of honey.
- Give him herb teas made from dillweed, dill seeds, or catnip.
- Have the child swallow crushed ice (only if he is old enough not to choke on it).
- Have him stick out his tongue and pull on it.
- Have him press lightly on his eyeballs.
- Press the cartilages just above the earhole on both ears (or have him do it).
- Have him tilt his chin toward his chest, and have someone press against the muscles in the middle of the back of his neck for several minutes.
- Put your thumb on one side and fingers on the other side of the big muscle that crosses from the back of the neck to the shoulder-tip, and grasp it firmly for several minutes.
- Rub the outer side of the lowest knuckle of the little finger.
- Apply pressure to the points on either side of the spine, just above the tips of the shoulder blades.
- Massage the soles of both feet, especially in the center.

HIVES

Hives (also called urticaria or nettle rash) are furiously itchy, raised red swollen spots with white centers. They can be as small as insect bites or as big as silver dollars, or may spread out together into large patches of misshapen puffiness.

A sudden outbreak of hives can be caused by an allergic reaction to a particular food (or overindulgence in it). Common triggers are shellfish, strawberries, nuts, eggs, milk, chocolate, pork, and wheat. Medications, such as aspirin or penicillin, can trigger hives. So can pollen, dust, insect bites (fleas produce a protein that can cause an allergic skin reaction; they don't even have to bite to do so), contact with certain metals (as in a bracelet, ring, or watchband), a reaction to extremes of heat or cold, a sensitivity to sunlight, or incompatible elements in blood transfusions. Anxiety, tension, and emotional stress can cause an attack.

Hives can last for a few hours, or a few weeks. The itching can be extremely uncomfortable and frightening, especially if the episode lasts a long time. Some people have only one case of hives in a lifetime; some have recurrent attacks. Rarely, the allergic reaction can be so severe that the swelling involves the throat and air passages and can interfere with breathing. If the child's throat feels swollen and breathing or swallowing are difficult, treat it as an emergency and get help right away. (See Emergencies chapter in Part Two; and ALLERGIES.)

WHAT A PHYSICIAN MAY DO

Most doctors prescribe antihistamine drugs to take away the misery. These medicines may relieve the itching and suppress the hives for a period of time; they usually need to be repeated every several hours until the body catches up and compensates for its allergic reaction. They do *not* remove the cause of the hives, and might prolong the attack. Some of the common antihistamines (such as Benadryl) can be bought without a prescription; a doctor may recommend them over the phone. Side effects of these drugs include drowsiness and digestive upsets. Also, some children experience symptoms of overdosage after taking only one or two of the regular doses; these include dry mouth, insomnia, apprehension, rapid heartbeat, pounding in the head, hallucinations, convulsions, fever, and breathing troubles. If the child is taking an antihistamine and has any of these symptoms, the medicine should be stopped instantly and never repeated.

If antihistamines don't control the symptoms, the doctor may prescribe corticosteroid drugs to be taken orally (applying them to the skin doesn't work). Again, these drugs are only removing the symptoms and may be interfering with the body's natural defenses—which means the hives may be more likely to recur or become chronic. Depending on the dose and the sensitivity of the child, corticosteroid drugs can interfere with hormonal balance, immune response, growth, and metabolism. Because of the dangers of drugs, conscientious parents should relieve a child's hives in other ways. If a child has frequent hives, his system needs to be brought into balance. (See ALLERGIES.)

If the condition is a true emergency that is threatening the child's breathing, a doctor will give an injection of epinephrine (adrenaline) to open the air passages; if this doesn't work, a tracheotomy (cutting an opening in the windpipe to make an artificial airway) may be performed and oxygen given.

WHAT YOU CAN DO AT HOME

PRACTICAL MEASURES AND NATURAL APPLICATIONS. Try to figure out the cause of the hives and remove it. Has a new food or drug been introduced? Has the child been exposed to chemicals—food additives, new clothing, a new shampoo or skin lotion? Do the hives break out after eating, after getting cold or wet, in a particular season, visiting relatives, after (or before) a test at school?

Have the child dress lightly; try to avoid anything that might cause her to sweat. Cold compresses or cool baths can soothe the itch and keep the swelling down. The juice of fresh chickweed is soothing if gently smoothed on the skin.

NUTRITION. Have the child eat foods to which you know she is not allergic. Give extra vitamin C, bioflavonoids, calcium, and pantothenic acid. These nutrients help the body produce its own antihistamine effect.

HOMEOPATHIC REMEDIES.
>
> *Apis mellifica.* Hives are intensely swollen, tender, itchy, may look bluish or have clear raised borders; often around eyes and mouth; worse from warmth, sweat, exercise, at night.
>
> *Arsenicum album.* Intense burning, and itching relieved by hot applications; hives may appear after overindulging in fruit; child may feel exhausted, afraid to be alone.
>
> *Dulcamara.* Hives come on from exposure to cold, damp; change to wet weather; stomach upset; better from warmth and moving around.
>
> *Ignatia* or *Natrum muriaticum.* Hives seem to be caused by emotional troubles.
>
> *Pulsatilla.* Hives come on after rich or unwholesome food, diarrhea; child is mild and weepy; worse from heat.
>
> *Rhus toxicodendron.* Worse from cold, wet, sweating; damp weather; scratching or rubbing brings out welts; oozing of clear fluid; itching relieved by hot water.

Urtica urens. Rash or large blotches; burns and itches like nettle stings; worse from heavy exercise; better from lying down. This remedy is good for hives caused by eating shellfish.

ACUPRESSURE AND MASSAGE.

LI 4: The point at the end of the crease between the thumb and index finger.

LI 11: A tender point at the thumb-side end of the elbow-crease when the arm is bent.

LV 3: A tender point midway between the first and second metatarsal bones.

IMPETIGO

Impetigo is a superficial but contagious skin disease involving staphlyococcus and streptococcus bacteria, that occurs when the skin's resistance is down. (Staph and strep bacteria can normally exist on healthy skin without causing infection.) Impetigo is seen mostly in warm or moist climates. First, little red pimples show up near the nostrils and lips (or, less frequently, on the scalp or arms and legs); then the pimples turn to blisters that eventually break and become raw red spots that do not hurt but ooze yellowish fluid and form a honey-colored crust. Sometimes swollen lymph nodes in the armpits, neck, or groin occur with impetigo near the areas of infection, especially if it is spreading. The infection is spread most readily by scratching.

Except for spreading, complications of impetigo are rare, but glomerulonephritis, a kidney inflammation caused by particular strains of strep bacteria, may occasionally follow an outbreak. The symptoms of glomerulonephritis are headache, nausea, loss of appetite, puffiness of the face and extremities, scanty, dark or bloody urine, and high blood pressure. If these symptoms occur, take the child to a doctor; occasionally this disease has dangerous consequences, but usually a child recovers quickly and completely.

WHAT A PHYSICIAN MAY DO
If the infection has spread severely, a thorough physical examination may be done to make sure no complications are developing. Most physicians prescribe antibiotic ointments; others believe

these do no good and may even slow healing. The doctor will advise you of methods of keeping the sores clean and preventing spreading.

WHAT YOU CAN DO AT HOME

PRACTICAL MEASURES AND NATURAL APPLICATIONS. Since impetigo is very contagious and it is almost impossible to keep a small child from touching the sores with her hands, it is important that you try to keep her out of situations in which she will touch other children. Any clothing, towels, washcloths, or bed linens that she has touched should be kept away from other people and washed and dried carefully. Make sure her fingernails are short and her hands are washed often. Wash *your* hands with soap and water right after you have touched the infected areas.

The crusts can be soaked off with warm water or compresses, and the sore spots washed with warm water and soap, or teas of the herbs calendula, comfrey, or echinacea. It is best to keep the areas exposed to air as much as possible, because this will speed healing (bacteria can stay alive beneath the crusts). However, if the sores are in an area that must be covered for some reason, wrap the part loosely with gauze, or tape on a large, thin pad of gauze. (Keep the tape well away from the infectious part, as it can damage the skin somewhat when torn off, and may make new openings for infection.) Tinctures of echinacea or calendula (diluted 5:1 with clean water) may be applied to the sores every few hours or used to soak the gauze.

NUTRITION. The child's diet should be free of refined and processed foods. Lots of fresh fruits and vegetables and good-quality protein should be eaten. Give him lots of fluid, especially vegetable juices. Nutritional supplements that help to raise the skin's resistance to infection are vitamins A, C, E, and zinc.

HERB TEAS. Red clover, echinacea, calendula, dandelion.

HOMEOPATHIC REMEDIES.
Arsenicum album. Sores are raw, dark; may ooze offensive pus; burning pains that are better from heat; child may be chilly, restless, anxious.
Antimonium crudum. Sores with crusts and oozing, may spread or run together; worse on the face; child may have white-coated tongue, dislike being looked at.

Dulcamara. Thick brown-yellow crusts that bleed on scratching; worse in cold, rainy weather.

Graphites. Scabs around the nose and mouth; sticky, honey-colored oozing; child may be overweight, glum, sensitive to music.

Hepar sulphuris calcareum. Sores very sore to touch, bleed easily; child may be sensitive to cold and drafts, irritable.

Mercurius vivus. Deep, open sores that ooze pus and blood; eruptions on face and head; child may drool, have swollen lymph nodes in the neck and bad breath.

Rhus toxicodendron. Clusters of sores; itching relieved by warm water; dark, clear oozing fluid; worse from cold and damp; child feels better in warm, dry weather and from moving around.

ACUPRESSURE AND MASSAGE.

ST 36: A tender point next to the outer side of the big bump at the top of the shin.

SP 6: A tender point three of the child's finger-breadths above the inner anklebone.

LU 1: A tender point in the indentation below the shoulder end of the collarbone.

LI 4: The point at the end of the crease between the thumb and index finger.

LI 11: A tender point at the thumb-side end of the elbow-crease when the arm is bent.

INDIGESTION AND GAS

Children are fascinated by burps and the other minor, noisy manifestations of gas—but sometimes gas overdoes it: stomachaches and gas pains are not much fun. A buildup of gas in the stomach or intestines can be caused by eating too quickly or too large a quantity, not chewing thoroughly enough, eating when excited or upset, swallowing air while talking, making animal noises, or singing at the table. Holidays, with much excitement and feasting, are likely occasions for internal upsets. Stresses such as parental conflict or divorce, moving, a new school, difficulties with studies, excitement about sports, music, love, or dramatics can turn the body's attention away from proper digestion.

Food allergy is often responsible for indigestion. Some children are overtly allergic to certain foods, but in addition, during times of stress or fatigue, a child may show an allergic reaction to certain foods or combinations of foods that are usually tolerated.

Most children's systems are capable of producing digestive enzymes and stomach acid sufficient for digestion. If these are supplied artificially (as they sometimes have to be to adults whose systems are more worn out and abused), their bodies respond by producing less. Therefore, digestive enzymes should not be given to children unless (as in diseases such as celiac disease or cystic fibrosis), the amount the body makes is so inadequate that help must come from outside.

WHAT A PHYSICIAN MAY DO

If a child has very distressing indigestion frequently, the doctor will give a physical examination and possibly order blood and urine tests to check for infections (such as colitis or appendicitis), anemia, or allergy. If she thinks it necessary, she may order barium X-ray studies to screen for ulcers or preulcerous conditions. She may also look for signs of tooth or gum disorders, poisoning or toxicity (from environmental chemicals, ingested nonfood substances, vitamin overdoses, etc.), or intestinal blockages caused by nervous tension, constipation, malposition of organs, or tumors. She may also do tests to check the functioning of the pancreas, liver, gallbladder, or kidneys.

If nothing serious is discovered, the doctor's advice will depend entirely on her orientation. Some doctors advise a natural, whole-foods diet; others advise bland, soft, starchy foods with little roughage, and over-the-counter antacids. Frequent use of antacids can upset the balance of minerals (especially magnesium) in the body; they may also induce the stomach to produce extra acid (a rebound effect) and thereby worsen digestion.

WHAT YOU CAN DO AT HOME

PRACTICAL MEASURES. Make sure your child eats meals in a relaxed, happy atmosphere and has plenty of time to dawdle. If he has trouble remembering to chew before swallowing, it might help to serve raw fruits or vegetables and meats cut up in small pieces. Tell a bolter or gulper that most of the food's taste is trapped inside it, and chewing is what brings it out. Although eating isn't everything, it can surely be regarded as a pleasant activity; parents should try to suspend tense topics at mealtime.

Give the child foods that he likes; choose those that are easy to digest and healthful. Yogurt, kefir, and cottage cheese are good sources of protein, unless the child has an allergy to cow's milk. Try goat's-milk products also. Children usually like fruit shakes or "smoothies" (fruits such as apples, bananas, oranges, or berries pureed in a blender, sometimes with yogurt), and sprouted grains in salads with tasty dressings. Raw vegetables can be marinated or sprinkled with lemon juice a few hours before eating to aid their digestion.

Because of their lack of fiber and nutrients, refined foods (white flour and sugar) and processed foods often stay too long in the intestines, and have time to putrefy and cause gas. Too much meat can do the same. Adding raw fruits, vegetables, and whole grains to the child's diet will help digestion move along before this can happen.

Do not give your child foods or combinations of foods that seem to bring on gas or stomachache. Common offenders are beans, peas, onions, bran, dried fruits, cooked cabbage, broccoli, cherries, even apples. Many gas-forming foods are very nutritious; you may find that they do not form gas if given at a different time of day, or by themselves rather than in combination—so, if the child likes them, experiment.

Beans seem to create less gas if they are soaked overnight, then rinsed and cooked in fresh water. Some people say that cooking them with an onion or clove of garlic, then throwing out the onion or garlic and water and rinsing off the beans, can take away the gassy properties; also try cooking them with mustard seeds or summer savory.

A combination of foods may cause a bad reaction even when the same foods used singly are easily digested. Many different systems for food combining have been publicized. Some say not to eat fruits and vegetables at the same meal; some say not to combine fruits and nuts; some say not to combine grains and proteins; others say you *should* combine them. Some say to eat all protein in the morning; others say eat only fruit till noon. Some authorities think that drinking fluids between meals, rather than during or near them, improves digestion because the digestive juices are not diluted by extra liquids. Others disagree. Like most other aspects of human health, food combination seems to be an individual matter. All you can do is experiment and see what works best for you and your child.

Papayas contain papain, an enzyme that is said to help the body digest protein. If you can't find the fresh fruit, look for papaya tablets in natural food stores.

Apple-cider vinegar—one teaspoon stirred into in a cup of water, hot or cold—can aid digestion. If the child wants it sweet, add a teaspoonful of honey. This should be given half an hour before meals.

B vitamins are especially good for controlling flatulence. Acidophilus culture, kelp, raw honey, and bee pollen added to the diet can also help.

Comfrey-pepsin tablets can help digestion; they are found in natural food stores. Chewing caraway, dill, or fennel seeds sometimes gives relief from indigestion. Activated charcoal capsules swallowed at bedtime or with meals may help reduce gas formation.

HERB TEAS. (A cup can be sipped slowly after a heavy meal, or during an attack of indigestion or gas pain.) Peppermint, spearmint, chamomile, ginger, alfalfa seed, blackberry, cinnamon, rose hips, thyme, catnip, dillweed, parsley, red clover, orange peel.

HOMEOPATHIC REMEDIES.

Arsenicum album. Burning, cramping pain; retching; child exhausted, anxious, chilly; after too much fruit, or spoiled things; worse from sight or smell of food.

Bryonia. Stomach feels heavy, sensitive to touch; bile or acid rises, tastes bitter or sour; worse from slightest motion; child is thirsty but drinks may cause nausea.

Carbo vegetabilis. Stomach and bowels fill with gas, no matter what food is eaten; meat, fats, and milk disagree; child bends double from pain; feels chilly, needs air.

Chamomilla. Stomach upset and crampy, sour or bitter vomiting; abdomen full of gas; diarrhea; child is angry, irritable; one or both cheeks flushed.

China. Feeling of weight and cold in stomach; gas seems stuck and won't move up or down; worse from fruit and milk; child is chilly; better from hard pressure, open air.

Colocynthis. Cramping, cutting pain relieved by hard pressure, doubling over, warmth; worse from drinking, or eating; may come on after indignation.

Ignatia. Cramping, sinking feeling in stomach; indigestion after emotional upset, grief, or loss; child is excitable, nervous, sighs, needs to breathe deeply; may crave indigestible or unusual foods and feel better from eating them.

Lycopodium. Pain and pressure in stomach; abdomen bloats after eating even a little; rumbling gas, worse from 4:00 to 8:00 P.M.; child craves sweets, likes warm drinks.

Magnesia phosphorica. Cramping in abdomen; retching, belching, bloating; indigestion preventing sleep; intense pain, better from warmth and rubbing; worse from eating.

Nux vomica. Pain and weight in stomach, sensitive to pressure; heartburn; after overindulging in strong or unhealthful foods; child is irritable, chilly; feels need to move the bowels or vomit, but can't.

Phosphorus. Burning pain, relieved by cold food and drink; belching, sour taste in mouth; child imaginative, animated, but easily tired; hungry soon after eating; worse from too much salt and from cold drinks growing warm in the stomach.

Pulsatilla. Pain, nausea, flatulence after rich foods; feels lump or pulsation in stomach; child hates fat but may crave butter; moody, clinging; worse in stuffy room.

ACUPRESSURE AND MASSAGE.

CV 12, 13: Tender points midway between the lower tip of the breastbone and the navel.

LI 4: The point at the end of the crease between the thumb and index finger.

ST 36: A tender point next to the outer side of the big bump at the top of the shin.

P 6: A point in the mid-forearm, three of the child's finger-breadths above the palm-side wrist-crease.

ST 25: The tender points two of the child's finger-breadths to either side of the navel.

INFECTIONS

Infection is a condition in which bacteria or viruses take hold in body tissues and produce toxic or inflammatory effects. Microorganisms are everywhere—in water, air, soil, on food, objects, animals; there is no escaping them. Many of the bacteria that cause infection (for instance, the common strains of staph and strep) are often harmlessly present in healthy people. Innumerable viruses and bacteria exist in the environment, and it takes poor immune function or low resistance to allow them to bring about infection.

The body's resistance to infection may be lowered by stresses such as wounds, inadequate cleanliness, poor nutrition, allergies, and emotional difficulties. It seems that certain individuals are more susceptible to particular sorts of infections and less affected by others. Some bacteria and viruses, however, are very potent disease agents and can make almost anyone ill.

Because of constant exposure, a person's system can build up resistance to familiar microorganisms in the environment. If a person not accustomed to these bacteria comes in contact with them, he or she may become infected. Traveler's diarrhea is an example of this: if a person from San Francisco goes to India and drinks the water, he may get quite sick; the same thing can happen if someone from India travels to San Francisco.

VIRUS-RELATED INFECTIONS

Most of the infectious illnesses children have are viral—colds and flus. Other virus-related troubles include: minor sore throats and earaches, conjunctivitis, croup, diarrhea, chicken pox, rubella, measles, mumps, and roseola. Herpes and "walking pneumonia" are also associated with viruses. Viral hepatitis and viral meningitis are serious viral infections. (See appropriate sections in this book.)

The more serious *complications* of viral diseases often involve bacteria that invade weakened tissues and cause infection. Bacterial complications that sometimes develop from common colds include ear infections, strep throat, and (rarely) kidney infection, pneumonia, and meningitis.

BACTERIAL INFECTIONS

When a cut or wound becomes infected, staph or strep bacteria are often involved, having taken hold because the damaged tissues have not been kept clean enough, or because the child's resistance is low. Signs of serious infection are: swelling around a wound (skin that is puffy and pink, or red, tight, hot, shiny); throbbing pain; fever; red streaks traveling outward from the edges of the wound; enlarged, tender lymph nodes; thick yellow or white discharge (pus).

Conditions seen in children involving bacteria include: infected eczema or diaper rash, impetigo, boils, acne, strep throat or tonsillitis, ear infection, mastoiditis, scarlet fever, kidney infection, rheumatic fever, pneumonia, and meningitis. (See appropriate sections in this book.)

WHAT A PHYSICIAN MAY DO
The doctor will examine the child, looking for signs of serious illness or complication. Antibiotics may be prescribed. Many physicians prescribe antibiotics for almost any infection, even viral ones, thinking that this serves to prevent potential complications. It is important for parents to know that these drugs do *not* work to support the child's immune system; they actually interfere with its function by poisoning and artificially removing the bacteria to which the body is trying to form immunity. This is why infections treated with antibiotics often come back soon after the course of medication has ended. Also, such drugs have many side effects and can cause severe allergic reactions. Antibiotics should be used only for serious bacterial infections and emergencies.

During an active infection, nutritionally oriented physicians may recommend giving vitamin C (50 to 500 mg every hour, depending upon the child's size and age) until the symptoms of infection begin to recede. Calcium, magnesium, and the B-complex vitamins are also used.

If a child has been hospitalized with serious infection, the parents have the right to demand intravenous administration of Vitamin C, B_6, and calcium to help the body fight infection and combat the toxic effects of any drugs that may be given. If this is what you want for your child, you will be more assured of getting it if you prepare ahead of time rather than waiting until you are in such a situation. Look for a nutritionally oriented physician who will endorse your request should the need arise.

WHAT YOU CAN DO AT HOME
PRACTICAL MEASURES. To prevent infections, children should be given a nourishing diet, plenty of rest, fresh air, and exercise, and

taught to keep themselves fairly (but not excessively) clean. Encourage the habits of washing the hands with soap and water after using the toilet; covering mouth and nose when coughing and sneezing; eating only clean food (for example, rewashing fruit that has fallen on the floor); and not sharing cups or utensils with other people or with animals.

Illnesses have varying periods of time during which they are contagious. Any child with a contagious illness should be kept away from other children until active signs of infection (such as fever, new eruptions, or discharge) are past—unless there is a particular reason for wanting other children to catch it (see CHICKEN POX, RUBELLA). The period between the time a child is exposed to a disease and the time the symptoms appear is called the incubation period. Incubation periods of different illnesses usually range from days to weeks.

The best treatment for any kind of infection is to strengthen the body's defenses. The child should have more rest than usual, be kept warm enough, have plenty of fresh air, nourishing food, and liquids.

NUTRITION. Make sure the child has plenty of fresh fruits and vegetables and high-quality protein to help with tissue repair and healing. Supplements that help combat both bacterial and viral infections are vitamins C, A, E, balanced B-complex, and zinc.

HERB TEAS. Echinacea, calendula, comfrey, garlic, lemon, rose hips.

HOMEOPATHIC REMEDIES. (See also FEVER, COLDS, FLU, BOILS, and other specific conditions.)

Aconitum napellus. Infections with sudden onset; child may be very anxious, thirsty; worse from cold wind and at night.

Belladonna. For conditions with intense heat, swelling, throbbing pain; worse from noise and jarring.

Bryonia. Infection with tearing pain, dry mouth, fever, chills; worse from motion, child wants to be left alone; better from pressure, keeping still, cold things.

Ferrum phosphoricum. For early stages of any infection or inflammation.

Hepar sulphuris calcareum. Infection with pus or discharge; child is irritable, sensitive, worse from drafts and cold; better from warmth and eating.

Mercurius vivus. Infectious states with swollen lymph nodes, foul breath; child may drool in sleep.

ACUPRESSURE AND MASSAGE.

ST 36: A tender point next to the outer side of the big bump at the top of the shin.

SP 6: A tender point three of the child's finger-breadths above the inner anklebone.

GV 14: The point at the tip of the big bump in the spine where the neck and upper back meet.

LI 4: The point at the end of the crease between the thumb and index finger.

LI 11: A tender point at the thumb-side end of the elbow-crease when the arm is bent.

LV 3: A tender point midway between the first and second metatarsal bones.

GB 20: A tender point in the muscles just below the base of the skull, midway between the central bump on the lower back of the head at the ear tip.

JAUNDICE

Jaundice is a condition in which the skin and the whites of the eyes have a yellowish tinge. It is not a disease in itself but a sign that the liver, for any of a number of reasons, is not converting and excreting the bile pigment bilirubin from the body.

In newborns, a little jaundice can be expected; several days may be needed for the newly functioning liver to catch up on its work. Any baby with jaundice however, should be evaluated by a doctor; too high a bilirubin level can mean something more serious. Jaundice in any child older than a newborn is rare and should always be evaluated by a physician. Jaundice may occur in hepatitis, anemia, allergic drug reactions, mononucleosis, or problems with the gallbladder or pancreas.

If the child's skin has yellow discoloration but the whites of her eyes do not, this may be a sign of carotenemia, a high carotene level in the blood. This is usually caused by a very high intake of carotene—as a supplement, in carrot juice, or from huge amounts of vegetables and fruits. Carotenemia is usually benign, but may occur with diabetes or thyroid problems.

WHAT A PHYSICIAN MAY DO

If a newborn infant looks very jaundiced, is lethargic, shows little interest in being fed, or vomits, a blood test will be performed. Causes of high bilirubin include blood-group incompatibility between mother and infant, infection, internal bleeding, diabetes or other metabolic problems (in the mother as well as the child), inability to take nourishment, or birth before full term.

A baby with a high bilirubin count may be kept in the hospital. Frequent feedings will be given, and the child exposed (with eyes protected) to measured levels of ultraviolet light. In extreme cases, where there is danger of kernicterus (a type of brain damage), exchange blood transfusion may be recommended.

When jaundice is present in children other than newborns, a doctor's treatment will depend on the cause. (See also ANEMIA and HEPATITIS.)

WHAT YOU CAN DO AT HOME

PRACTICAL MEASURES. If jaundice is very mild in a newborn, give the infant frequent feedings and extra fluids to help the intestines move the extra bile out more speedily. Bringing the baby into daylight for moderate periods several times a day may help to clear jaundice, but avoid direct sunlight and overheating.

Since jaundice is only a symptom, its cause should be detected and the child treated accordingly. The following general measures may help to strengthen the liver. (For homeopathic remedies, see HEPATITIS and ANEMIA.)

NUTRITION. The child should have a pure diet including lots of pure water, fruit and vegetable juices, and herb teas, as well as raw fruits and vegetables, whole grains and good-quality protein (especially fertile eggs). Oats, barley, onions, garlic, carrots, beets, radishes, parsley, pears, apples, and lemons are particularly good foods in such cases. Do not give any fatty or fried foods, so that the child's system may cleanse itself and rest.

Supplements of vitamins A, C, D, E, B-complex (especially B_6 and pantothenic acid), calcium, magnesium, and lecithin are beneficial.

HERB TEAS. Peppermint, rose hips, fennel, dandelion, chicory.

ACUPRESSURE AND MASSAGE.

LV 14: A tender point on the front of the rib cage, midway between the nipple and the lower ribs.

LV 3: A tender point midway between the first and second metatarsal bones.

LI 4: The point at the end of the crease between the thumb and index finger.

JOINT CONDITIONS

A joint is the place where two bones meet, and the space between them; most are held together by connective tissue, stabilized by muscles. Some contain fluid. Joint pains in children are usually caused by injuries such as sprained thumbs and turned ankles. Children's joints may hurt from overexertion in play or sports; the soreness may not be noticed until hours or days after the activity. Arthritis, more serious inflammation of the joints, is very rare in children. If it does occur, it is usually part of an illness like rheumatic fever, sickle cell anemia, or rubella. Muscle and bone pains are often experienced during viral illnesses like colds and flu. Occasionally, rheumatoid arthritis may be diagnosed in a child. Food allergy may also be a cause of joint pain.

"Growing pains" are not felt in the joints but in the muscles and tendons of the legs. For instance, the child's leg may hurt when *he* moves it, but not if it is raised and moved by someone else. Growing pains are often felt at night, and may correspond with growth spurts.

In athletic adolescent boys, swelling and tenderness of the knee, made worse by exercise, may indicate Osgood-Schlatter disease. This is a condition in which bone formation in the tibial tuberosity (the bump below the knee, to which large muscles attach) is irregular. This is not dangerous, though often uncomfortable.

Joint pains in children may be caused by misalignments of bones of the spine, pelvis, legs, feet, shoulders, arms, or wrists.

Even if misalignment is slight, it can lead to unbalanced muscular development throughout the child's frame, which may put abnormal strain on the joints. Often the area in which pain is felt is not the area of true misalignment: the sore part may be trying to compensate. If your child has posture problems or long-lasting joint pains that seem to have no other cause, find a chiropractor who is very gentle and experienced in treating children, to restore correct alignment and prescribe appropriate exercise.

WHAT A PHYSICIAN MAY DO

A doctor will examine the joint and assess it for injury, infection, or arthritis. If a fracture is suspected, an X ray may be taken. Sometimes a needle is inserted into the joint capsule to remove fluid to check for bleeding or infection. Damaged ligaments and cartilage may need surgical repair.

Drugs such as cortisone are sometimes given to reduce inflammation. These can interfere with growth and hormonal balance, and children should not take them.

WHAT YOU CAN DO AT HOME

PRACTICAL MEASURES AND NUTRITION. If the joints are inflamed and tender as part of a viral illness or infection, see COLDS, FLU, and RUBELLA.

Joint pain from a new injury (sprain or strain) should be treated by applying ice packs (five minutes on, ten minutes off, repeated several times). Do not use heat. Ice can increase circulation and thereby speed healing without increasing the swelling. If the injury is more than forty-eight hours old, heat may be helpful to relax tight muscles. Calcium, magnesium, and vitamin C are good for reducing pain and inflammation in such injuries. Homeopathic remedies (see below) often diminish pain and speed recovery.

Poultices of comfrey leaves, or cloths soaked with castor oil and placed on the painful areas for half an hour, may help soothe inflamed or injured joints. *Arnica* ointment or oil may be rubbed on the sore parts, if the skin is not broken.

Growing pains respond to good nutrition, massage, and moderate exercise. (See also Homeopathic Remedies, below.) Good nutrition, rest—and avoiding athletics for several weeks or months—will help with Osgood-Schlatter disease.

Any child with painful or swollen joints should have plenty of high-quality protein, whole grains such as rice and millet, and fresh fruits and vegetables (especially sour cherries, bananas, apples, pineapple, green beans, potatoes, celery, yams, parsley, garlic, and alfalfa sprouts). Dairy products and wheat may cause joint irritation; if your child eats them, watch for an aggravation of symptoms. Allergies to other foods may also contribute (see ALLERGIES).

If the family has a history of rheumatoid arthritis, joint soreness may be helped by avoiding tomatoes, peppers, and eggplant (all members of the nightshade family).

Vitamins C, E, B-complex (including pantothenic acid and niacin or niacinamide), calcium, magnesium, cod-liver oil, alfalfa tablets, kelp, and papaya-bromelain tablets (taken with meals) may be beneficial. Make sure the child has adequate vitamin D and gets plenty of sunshine (but watch for burning).

HERB TEAS. Parsley, comfrey, nettle, fresh cornsilk, cider vinegar and honey, thyme; oatstraw tea (a teaspoonful per cup of water, boiled half an hour) may be drunk or added to the bath.

HOMEOPATHIC REMEDIES.
> *Arnica montana.* For new sprains and strains with lots of swelling and bruising; also for bruised sensation in uninjured joints; other remedies may follow it.
> *Bryonia.* Sharp pain on the slightest motion, worse as motion continues.
> *Ledum palustre.* Joint feels numb or cold, but is better from ice or cold soaking.
> *Rhus toxicodendron.* Pain and stiffness of joints, better with warmth and continued motion.
> *Ruta graveolens.* Sprains or bruised bone coverings, pulled or torn ligaments.
> *Symphytum.* Bad sprains, especially if other remedies do not work deeply.

ACUPRESSURE AND MASSAGE.
> BL 60: A tender point in the hollow behind the outer anklebone in front of the Achilles tendon.

BL 11: The points in the muscles two of the child's thumb-widths to the sides of the vertebra below the big bump at the base of the neck.

LI 4: The point at the end of the crease between the thumb and index finger.

LV 3: A tender point midway between the first and second metatarsal bones.

LI 20: The tender points where the creases of the cheek meet the nose.

LYMPH NODES

The phrase *swollen glands* is usually used to refer to swollen lymph nodes (although glands do swell: mumps causes swollen salivary glands). Lymph nodes play a part in immune function, and groups of them are located in different parts of the body, including the neck, armpits, groin, and abdomen. Normal lymph nodes are more prominent in some children than in others; children who catch many colds or are physically run-down may have chronically swollen lymph nodes. If lymph nodes in a particular part of the body are swollen, it is likely that there is infection near that area. Such infection may be caused by viral diseases (e.g., colds, sore throats, conjunctivitis, roseola), bacterial diseases (e.g., ear infection, strep throat, scarlet fever), infected wounds, and scratches or bites from animals or insects. Swollen lymph nodes at the back of the neck and skull often accompany rubella (German measles) and mononucleosis. Rarer, more serious conditions such as leukemia and Hodgkin's disease include swollen lymph nodes among their symptoms.

WHAT A PHYSICIAN MAY DO
The doctor's diagnostic measures and treatment will depend on the child's other symptoms. Probably a thorough physical examination will be given, and blood tests run if the source of the infection is not obvious.

WHAT YOU CAN DO AT HOME
PRACTICAL MEASURES. Since lymph nodes become enlarged while the body is fighting many kinds of infection, the cause of the child's specific problem has to be found and treated. Remember

that nodes usually swell near the area of infection. Consider any of the conditions listed above that might apply, and refer to the appropriate sections of this book. If the swelling is severe and painful or the child feels really sick, check with a doctor.

For nutrition, herbs, homeopathic remedies, and acupressure points, see INFECTIONS; see also sections on specific conditions.

Measles (Rubeola)

Measles is a very contagious viral disease. Its early symptoms resemble a bad cold—weakness, runny nose, mild fever, dry or hacking cough. The child's eyes will usually be red and watery and very sensitive to light. Over the next few days, the fever may gradually rise, rather than falling as you would expect in a cold. On the inner surface of the cheeks next to the molars, little white spots that look like grains of salt (called Koplik's spots) show up. On the fourth or fifth day of illness, the fever might go down a little, and Koplik's spots fade as a blotchy, pink, flat or slightly raised rash comes out on the face and neck and behind the ears. The blotches spread quickly and run together, covering the chest and abdomen and, later, the arms and legs. The rash eventually turns brownish. By the time a week is up, the child has usually begun to feel better. A child with measles is contagious from two to four days before the rash appears and all through the illness.

Measles can have complications; sore throats, ear infections, and pneumonia (especially in infants) are common. Rarely, an infection of the brain (measles encephalitis) occurs, with high fever, convulsions, and coma; this may be of short duration, with recovery within a week, but it has been known to lead to central nervous system damage, or even death. A severe, pounding headache, dark, dry tongue and lips, purple or black rash, vomiting and diarrhea, difficult breathing, any unusual bleeding, loss of consciousness, and delirium are danger signs. See a doctor immediately.

WHAT A PHYSICIAN MAY DO
Because measles is so contagious, in uncomplicated cases it is best not to take the child to a doctor's office. Telephone if you need advice.

If the child's eyes become badly inflamed, the doctor may prescribe a lotion to soothe them. Some doctors give phenolated calamine lotion for an itchy rash.

For cases with complications such as encephalitis, a doctor may put the child in the hospital, give antibiotic drugs and possibly measles immune serum globulin.

If a child has been exposed to measles but has not yet come down with it, and is very run-down or seems to be at risk for complications because of past illnesses, gamma globulin can be given to prevent or lessen the disease.

WHAT YOU CAN DO AT HOME

PRACTICAL MEASURES. Keep the measled child away from other children who have not had it yet, in bed, in a room that is well ventilated and not too brightly lit. Give him plenty to drink so he doesn't become dehydrated. If it feels nice to him, sponge his face and hands with cool water. Baths with sage tea added may soothe itching.

NUTRITION. Don't make him eat if he doesn't want to; if he does, try things like oatmeal, barley soups, and bananas. Give plenty of fluid, teas, and juices, extra vitamins C, A, E, and zinc are also beneficial.

HERB TEAS. Peppermint, echinacea, elder flower, slippery elm, ginger, flaxseed.

HOMEOPATHIC REMEDIES. (See also FEVER.)

Aconitum napellus. If illness came on suddenly with violent fever, child is agitated and has eye pain in the light; give in the early stages of measles.

Belladonna. Child has a red face, throbbing headache, sore throat, restless, worse with noise and light; may become delirious.

Bryonia. If rash is slow in appearing or not well-developed; congestion in the chest and painful cough; muscles ache; child wants to lie still and not be disturbed.

Euphrasia. Eyes very red, swollen, streaming, very sensitive to light; tears may irritate the face; headache, runny nose.

Gelsemium. Child is very droopy and lethargic, has chills with fever, aches, and has an itchy rash.

Kali bichromium. Cold symptoms worsen as illness goes on; hoarse sore throat, sticky eyes, rattling cough, earache; long, tough, stringy mucus.

Pulsatilla. Cold symptoms are prominent and rash is slow to develop; child may be clinging or weepy, feels worse at sundown.

Rhus toxicodendron. Rash is very itchy, oozing fluid; better from warm bathing; worse at night.

For acupressure points, see FEVER.

MENINGITIS

Meningitis is an extremely serious disease, far too dangerous to treat at home. It sometimes occurs in epidemics (at which time it is very infectious, both to children and adults), or it may follow as a complication of illnesses such as middle-ear infection, tonsillitis, measles, mumps, polio, and tuberculosis. Infection—which may be related to bacteria, viruses, or fungus—travels from other parts of the body through the bloodstream to the meninges—the coverings of the brain and spinal cord—to cause this extreme illness.

Symptoms of meningitis may begin mildly, with sore throat, runny nose, and low fever, but as the infection progresses the fever soars, the neck and back become so stiff it is hard for the child to touch her chin to her chest or bend to put her head between her knees, headache becomes excruciating, and there may be extreme irritability, vomiting, and stupor. Sometimes a red or purplish rash (made up of small points of bleeding under the skin) comes out all over the body.

In babies and children younger than two, symptoms may be different: fever, vomiting, high-pitched crying, irritability, tight or bulging fontanels (the soft spots on the skull), possibly even convulsions. Often the neck is not stiff.

WHAT A PHYSICIAN MAY DO
A sample of spinal fluid will be taken, to determine the agent (usually bacterial or viral) that has brought on the infection. Specific medication will be given accordingly. Dehydration and electrolyte

imbalances may be kept under control intravenously. Some doctors administer high doses of vitamin C—several grams per hour—intravenously, along with conventional drug therapy. Vitamin C helps to support immune function and counteract toxicity from drugs. In an emergency, it may be difficult to locate a doctor who will authorize this, but if you have already checked around, you will be prepared in case of such an emergency. You have a right to ask for such therapies in the hospital, but health professionals have many different attitudes, and the extent to which the patient's rights are honored varies widely from doctor to doctor and hospital to hospital.

WHAT YOU CAN DO AT HOME

If a child shows signs of meningitis, it is an emergency and a doctor's help should be sought immediately. Some forms of meningitis can be fatal or extremely damaging. The home care measures mentioned here are in no way meant to replace the help of a physician; they are not cures, and are suggested only for cases in which there is absolutely no chance of getting professional help.

Keep the child in bed in a darkened room with good ventilation and no visitors except the person caring for him. (Try to have people take shifts staying with the sick child; he should never be left alone.)

Give gentle massage and apply a warm damp cloth to abdomen and lower spine.

One procedure used to draw out inflammation, recommended by a naturally oriented physician: Dissolve several tablespoons of epsom salts in a bowl of warm water; let the back of the patient's head rest in the bowl for as long as it is comfortable to do so; repeat this frequently.

NUTRITION. If the child is conscious, have him drink plenty of fluids—water, fruit juices, vegetable and barley broths. This will prevent dehydration and help cleanse his system. Give as much vitamin C as possible; mix it into drinks if necessary.

HERB TEAS. Echinacea, comfrey, catnip, red clover, goldenseal.

For homeopathic remedies, see FEVER and INFECTIONS.

ACUPRESSURE AND MASSAGE. (See also FEVER.)
- Rub the top side of the lower knuckle of the thumb, and the outer side of the middle knuckle of the little finger.
- If the child can bear the touch, gently massage the whole ear, especially along the curved ridge in the middle, and the uppermost portion of the lobe.

    ST 36: A tender point next to the outer side of the big bump at the top of the shin.

    SP 6: A tender point three of the child's finger-breadths above the inner anklebone.

CAUTION: Although the above procedures may be valuable in combating meningitis, remember that it is an *extremely dangerous* disease, and medical care must be obtained as soon as is humanly possible.

MENSTRUAL PROBLEMS

Menstrual periods usually begin in girls between the ages of ten and sixteen. The flow may be heavy or light and last from several days to a week. The interval between the first day of each period is usually about a month, although a normal cycle varies from person to person.

Some girls look forward to the transition from childhood to puberty, and take the first period in stride. For others there is some embarrassment, fear, or emotional conflict. Emotional support and accurate information about the hormonal and sexual changes in her body are important for a child at such a time, along with respect for her privacy. Moodiness should definitely be tolerated. She should be welcomed to talk over feelings, questions, and problems, and not be made to feel self-conscious or threatened in any way.

Fatigue, irritability, water retention, craving for sweets, headache, acne, breast tenderness, low back pain, and cramping may accompany menstrual periods in some degree. Such symptoms may be caused in part by nutritional deficiencies, lack of exercise, spinal or muscular problems, inefficiency of the liver in breaking down hormones, or hereditary tendencies. Many have a strong emotional component.

If a girl has very painful periods, heavy bleeding, very irregular periods, periods that begin at a very early age, or does not have her first period by the age of sixteen (unless there is a family history of this), she should see a sympathetic, experienced physician with whom it is easy for her to talk. Teenagers who are sexually active, or have problems they find hard to bring up with their parents, may need an opportunity to talk frankly to someone besides their parents. A friendly woman doctor is usually the best person for a teenage girl to work with: she will know from experience what it is like to have a female body—something the best-intentioned of men can only guess.

WHAT A PHYSICIAN MAY DO

Depending upon the symptoms, the doctor may check for structural problems, malposition of the uterus, adhesions, growths, cysts, hormonal problems, as well as thyroid imbalance, diabetes, malnutrition, weight problems, infections, drug use, emotional difficulties, or pregnancy. If necessary, the uterus may be repositioned through gentle manipulation. Hormones, surgery, or medications such as diuretics (which can upset water and mineral balance), tranquilizers, muscle relaxants, and analgesics (which may cause drowsiness, dizziness, weakness, internal bleeding, liver damage, or be addictive) are sometimes recommended to remove the symptoms. Over-the-counter medications may also have harmful side effects. Help your child avoid all drugs: all they do is mask or alter symptoms; none corrects the problem. Provide your child with natural therapies; explain that these work to correct the way her body functions and can eventually bring permanent relief. Constitutional homeopathy, acupuncture, herbal therapy, nutrition, yoga or exercise programs, spinal and cranial adjustments, and counseling are often successful in correcting menstrual problems without the use of invasive therapies, hormones, or drugs. Look for experienced, sympathetic practitioners.

TOXIC SHOCK SYNDROME

Toxic shock syndrome is a very serious condition related to toxin-producing strains of staphylococcus bacteria. It seems to occur more frequently in teenage girls and women under thirty who are using tampons than in other members of the population. (The estimated number is 1 to 17 cases per 100,000 menstruating girls and women each year.) The early symptoms include sudden high fever, vomiting, fainting, dizziness, sore throat, and a rash that looks like sunburn. Such symptoms may also occur with flu or other illness, but if they occur during menstruation and a girl is using tampons, the tampon should be removed and a doctor consulted right away. To reduce the likelihood of toxic shock occurring, lower-absorbency tampons should be used and changed often; whenever possible, especially at night or on days of lighter flow, pads should be used instead of tampons. (See also INFECTIONS.)

WHAT YOU CAN DO AT HOME

PRACTICAL MEASURES. Massage and tension-relieving techniques are helpful to some girls and women with menstrual problems. Deep breathing exercises, simple yoga stretches, knee-to-chest or pelvic rocking exercises also help. A warm bath with sage or lavender added, or a hot water bottle on the abdomen, may be soothing. Snuggling under the covers with a book is sometimes enough to ease discomfort and cramping. Regular daily exercise in a pleasant form such as dancing, bicycling, or active sports will help a child's periods become less troublesome. Very heavy exercise and strenuous running are not recommended for girls with menstrual problems.

NUTRITION. Premenstrual tension and pain during periods can be reduced by eating plenty of fresh fruits and vegetables and avoiding sweets, refined and processed foods, and foods with additives. Fried foods, cheese, chocolate, butter, margarine, shortening, and red meat should not be eaten in large amounts as they can make the liver's job of dealing with shifting hormones and cleansing the blood more difficult. High-quality protein from fish, poultry, or vegetable sources, whole grains, kelp, sesame, flax, and sunflower seeds may all be helpful.

A balanced multivitamin and mineral supplement, along with extra vitamin E (400–600 IU per day), vitamin C, balanced B-complex (especially B_6), magnesium, and calcium can help prevent premenstrual tension, bloating, breast swelling and tenderness, and menstrual cramps. Craving sweets may signify a need for protein or iron; craving chocolate is often a sign of a need for magnesium.

HERB TEAS. Red raspberry leaf, chamomile, hops, nettle, garlic.

HOMEOPATHIC REMEDIES.

Belladonna. Bright red flow; sudden, intense pain, weight and pressure in pelvic organs; worse from motion, jarring, walking, bending over; better sitting up straight.

Caulophyllum. Pains worst before period starts, pain darts to other areas; profuse flow, back pain, dizziness.

Chamomilla. Pains like labor pains, intense cramping; extreme irritability, anger; relief from warmth but worse from being hot; worse from open air, wind, and at night.

Cimicifuga. Irregular periods; pains cause doubling over, stab from side to side; low back pain; nervousness, depression, a feeling of being "inside a dark cloud."

Cocculus. Periods with lots of dark flow; pressing uterine pain, hemorrhoids; weakness, dizziness, nausea; child is sensitive, worse from loss of sleep.

Colocynthis. Cramping relieved by hard pressure on abdomen, curling up, or bending double; burning pain near ovaries; worse after anger or indignation.

Ignatia. Spasmodic pains in abdomen, sudden weakness; contradictory symptoms (child may be chilled but want cold drinks, feel nauseous but want to eat strong foods, etc.); worse from emotional upset, anger injustice, grief.

Magnesia phosphorica. Intense cramping relieved by warmth and pressure.

Nux vomica. Irregular periods, often early; cramping pain extending to low back and pelvic bones, often with urge to move the bowels; chilly, irritable, pushy.

Pulsatilla. Pain, faintness, dizziness, nausea; moodiness with tears.

Veratrum album. Periods too early, profuse flow that exhausts her; cold sweat, fainting, vomiting and diarrhea; child may be sad, sullen, precocious.

ACUPRESSURE AND MASSAGE.

SP 6: A tender point three of the child's finger-breadths above the inner anklebone.

CV 3, 4, 5: Points in the midline of the abdomen, between pubic bone and navel.

BL 47: A point in the muscles of the back just above the level of the ridge at the top of the pelvis.

SP 2: A point on the inner side of the foot at the big toe joint.

KI 3: The tender point just behind the upper rear aspect of the inner anklebone.

MENTAL, EMOTIONAL, AND BEHAVIORAL PROBLEMS

A child's health is greatly affected by his mental and emotional balance and his ability to deal with stresses when they arise. A child's physical health can also affect his frame of mind and emotions. While this book cannot attempt to solve deep or complicated problems, the following practical measures, dietary changes, and natural remedies may ease tension and help some children through the ups and down of life. Minor emotional upsets are normal, of course, and should only be "treated" with love and understanding, not with medicine.

Children may naturally become anxious for many reasons: school pressures; self-consciousness or problems with confidence; moving or changing schools; a new baby in the family; family troubles such as alcoholism, parental conflict, or separation; real or imagined pressures from parents or siblings; death of a loved one or relative. These are all real stresses that may be hard for a child to handle. A child's difficulty in dealing with anxiety may be expressed in the form of bedwetting, behavior problems, stomachaches and other digestive disorders, hyperventilation, asthma, headaches, problems with eating or sleeping, and depression or withdrawal.

WHAT A PROFESSIONAL MAY DO

When parents or teachers find themselves unable to cope with a child's problems, family therapy or counseling can be very useful. As with all other types of encounters with physicians or professionals, parents should be involved in the process, and must make an effort to find a counselor whom they trust and whose approach agrees with them (and especially agrees with the child). There are many different approaches to therapy; the attitudes held by public mental health workers, psychotherapists, social workers, and psychiatrists can vary tremendously. Some practitioners require that the entire family be involved in working out problems; some see the child alone; some use play therapy, art therapy, and other methods; some are strongly inclined toward the use of medications. Parents should not close their minds to therapy when long-standing or serious problems arise, but they must also use caution: the benefits derived from psychological treatment depend entirely upon its suitability to the child's personality and needs. Some children subjected to psychiatric evaluation and treatment experience an increase in anxiety and begin to form an image of themselves as disturbed. Psychoactive or antidepressant medications rarely solve problems; they're far more likely to cover them up. Remember that the goal of any sort of health care is not to *establish* a problem, but to relieve it, so the child regains his health.

WHAT YOU CAN DO AT HOME

PRACTICAL MEASURES. Make the child feel welcome to tell you her feelings, and acknowledge them: do not tell her they are wrong or make her feel judged. Try not to overreact or feel threatened by feelings you may not understand or approve of. If the way she expresses her feelings is inappropriate (causing pain or irritation to others, or damage to objects), help her find healthier ways of venting frustration such as active sports, jumping rope, riding a bike, harmless "violence" such as pounding on pillows; finding a place to yell or scream where it doesn't bother other people; drawing or painting pictures, writing stories, or acting out dramas to deal with fears and conflicts.

If there are serious problems in the family, be honest about them; do not cover them up or encourage the child to deny that they exist. They may be frightening to you, too; no one's fear will be relieved by suppressing it, and no problem will be solved by pretending there is no problem.

Make the child feel loved and accepted. Listen to him, hug him, find things for him to do that make him feel comfortable, interested, and happy. Do not impose your idea of what a child should be doing, thinking, or feeling; he is an individual. Help him find his own talents and good points, and (without pressure) give him opportunities to develop them. Do not forget that, even though they are smaller and less mature, children are just as complicated and individual as adults are.

Good physical health can help a child handle stress. Children with allergies, blood-sugar problems, or endocrine imbalances may have mental or emotional problems that are manageable once the physical disorders are overcome. Good nutrition, adequate sleep, fresh air, exercise, and opportunities for having fun are vital for reducing the effects of stress.

NUTRITION. The child should have a nourishing diet, free of all refined flours and sugars, processed foods, artificial sweeteners, or foods containing caffeine, coloring, or additives. The standard American diet has been linked with behavioral problems in children. (See Nutrition chapter in Part One.)

A good multivitamin and mineral supplement, extra B-complex (including niacin and pantothenic acid), vitamins C, E, calcium, magnesium, zinc, beta carotene, and essential fatty acids (found in cold-pressed oils such as sunflower) may be helpful.

HOMEOPATHIC REMEDIES. *NOTE:* If a child has deep or serious problems, or if indications for one particular remedy are not clear, do not attempt to choose a remedy yourself. Take the child to see an experienced prescriber.

Aconitum napellus. Extreme fear and anxiety, even from apparently trivial causes; heart palpitations; numb, tingling feet and hands; better from being in fresh air (though worse from cold wind); child is thirsty; worse at night, in warm rooms, worse from music.

Antimonium crudum. Child is very contradictory, cries, sulks, can't bear to be looked at or touched.

Argentum nitricum. Very nervous and impulsive; may be hyperactive; can become very fearful, often getting diarrhea when anticipating some stressful situation; fear of being alone; may have delusions, such as thinking houses are going to fall down on him, or strange impulses, such as the urge to jump out the window; craves sweets and salt.

Arsenicum album. Great anguish and fear; child cannot be left alone; oversensitive to everything; hates disorder; nervous, congestive headaches; asthma; very irritable and restless, but exertion may cause great exhaustion; frightening dreams of fire, danger, evil; hallucinations (thinks she sees burglars or beasts in her room); fear of death; worse after midnight and in wet weather; better from warmth, having head propped up, warm drinks.

Baryta carbonica. Child may be a slow learner, very forgetful, or backward in physical development; excessively shy, hides from people; does not seem to be interested in much and sits around listlessly; worse after eating, better after walking.

Belladonna. Child may be very intense and outgoing; may wake in the night in terror; can have fits of extreme fear, delirium, hallucinations (ghosts, monsters, horrible faces, big black dogs); feels driven to escape, bite, cry out; these episodes may alternate with times of seeming quite all right.

Borax. Child may be quite capable of learning but seems to prefer not to try; very startled by sudden noises; is terrified of falling (dreads elevators, stairs, swings, any downward motion); child may be bad-humored and lethargic before a bowel movement, and quite cheerful afterward.

Calcarea carbonica. Child may be flabby or fat, cold, sweaty; very stubborn; not energetic, but restless and anxious, especially in the evening and night; awful dreams and visions of terrible faces; may eat chalk, pencil leads, etc.; craves eggs, salt; likes ice cream but often has a bad reaction to milk.

Calcarea phosphorica. Child may be skinny, with growing pains, cold hands and feet; headaches during or after school; colic and gas; often acts peevish or miserable; craves bacon and sausages; worse in cold, damp weather; better when warm and dry.

Chamomilla. Child is extremely irritable and angry; screams and hurls things, even if she has just asked for them; unstable; hits people, stamps her feet; pains in the stomach, head, and teeth—all pains seem intolerable, drive her frantic; better from being carried and distracted with something new.

Cina. Child is very bad-humored, kicks and hits; his body stiffens with anger; after an initial irritable outburst, he can usually be calmed by being held and rocked; the child may pick his nose frequently, have headaches, stomachaches, worms; worse at night and from too much heat or sun.

Fluoric acid. Child may be very energetic and enjoy life, but can develop violent, unreasoning dislikes to certain other children; may become tired or headachy from concentrating at school, or from having to wait too long to urinate; he may need frequent snacks to keep from becoming ill; may have sweaty feet and hands, red cracked tongue, teeth that rot at the roots for no apparent reason.

Gelsemium. Child may be depressed and lethargic, nervous and fearful at upcoming stress; "stage fright;" diarrhea, headache, achy muscles, fear of falling.

Hyoscyamus. Child very jealous, resentful of a sibling or step-parent; very talkative; may take off clothes or urinate or defecate in inappropriate situations.

Ignatia. Hysterical, fearful, sad, or depressed, has mood swings; tobacco smoke can cause sickness; may feel better after eating peculiar things; after emotional shock, grief, extended strain.

Lycopodium. Child may seem overstressed mentally, look or act too "old"; may lack confidence but be haughty or domineering to-ward younger children yet shy or cowardly with older ones; tear-ful, apprehensive, irritable; may have gas, digestive problems; worse from 4:00 to 8:00 P.M.

Nux vomica. Very irritable, oversensitive, sentimental, angry, tense, annoyed by trifles, "driven"; may be hyperactive; desires spicy foods and sweets; chilly; constipated; may have difficulty sleeping.

Stramonium. May be violent, very suspicious of others, with reac-tions out of proportion to the circumstances; may have nightmares or awake in the night screaming; fears of darkness, tunnels, water—especially being submerged or having water poured over her head (as in washing hair or taking showers).

Veratrum album. May be very precocious, possibly arrogant, or isolated, feeling hurt that his superiority or intelligence is not rec-ognized; chilly, clammy, pale; worse at night; better from warmth and walking.

HERB TEAS. Chamomile, peppermint, hops, small amounts of sage.

ACUPRESSURE AND MASSAGE.

    HT 3: A tender point on top of the bony bump on the little-finger side of the elbow, at end of crease when the arm is bent.

·   Rub or press firmly on the point at the inner edge of the wrist crease (palm and little-finger side).

- Massage (or have the child rub) all tender points along the sternum ('breastbone').
- Find the bumps (which may be tender) on either side of the notch at the base of the throat, where the collarbone and breastbone meet. Hold or rub one of these points with the tip of your left index finger, while applying gentle pressure to the child's navel with your right thumb. After about a minute, move your left index finger to the point on the other side, still touching the navel with your right thumb, and hold for another minute or so.
- Give your child frequent relaxing backrubs and neckrubs if he likes them.

Specially trained chiropractors, osteopaths, and craniosacral therapists perform gentle manipulations of the cranial bones and spinal column; this has often been helpful to children with emotional or behavior problems.

MOTION SICKNESS

Many children are prone to motion sickness—nausea or dizziness while riding in a car, bus, boat, airplane, swing, merry-go-round, or carnival ride. This is apparently caused when the child's vision and position perception are not compatible with the movement of the vehicle: this upsets the balance mechanism in the inner ear and the child feels very ill. Signs of impending motion sickness are: abrupt silence in the middle of normal riding-in-the-car chatter, sleepiness or dizziness, pallor, whining, tears, sweating and salivation. Susceptibility to motion sickness seems to peak in mid-childhood and decrease with adolescence. This may be partly because increased height allows the child, even when sitting in the back of a vehicle, to look forward through the windshield rather than sideways, and possibly because of a greater capacity for concentration.

WHAT A PHYSICIAN MAY DO
Doctors sometimes recommend antihistamines to control motion sickness, but parents should remember that these drugs (even the over-the-counter ones) have side effects. It is possible at any time

for a child to have a severe reaction to a drug, or to develop an allergy to it. Using drugs for trivial ailments is foolish, and possibly deadly.

WHAT YOU CAN DO

PRACTICAL MEASURES AND NUTRITION. If possible, let the child ride in the front seat. Having a window rolled down for fresh air is usually helpful. If a child is assured that, should she feel nauseous, all she has to do is say so and the driver will find a place to pull over, the removal of anxiety may decrease her chance of becoming carsick.

Ask the child not to read in the car or play games that require looking down. Play guessing games or talk together for amusement, encouraging the child to relax and continue looking straight ahead.

Motion sickness is often worse when the blood sugar is low, so giving your child a light, easily digested meal before traveling is a good idea. B-vitamin supplements taken just before a trip are also recommended. Crackers and ice water (from a thermos) can be brought along, to keep the child's insides steady.

HERB TEAS. (Carry them in a thermos, or serve them before, or after, a trip.) Ginger root, fennel, orange peel, basil, peppermint, raspberry leaf.

HOMEOPATHIC REMEDIES.

Argentum nitricum. Nausea, retching; anxiety, faintness, trembling, perception and sense of balance may be disturbed; child is imaginative, craves sweets, salt.

Arsenicum album. Nausea, worse from sight or smell of food; vomits bile and mucus; burning pain; child chilly, restless but exhausted; thirsty, drinks in sips.

Borax. Nausea, pain, gas, diarrhea; child has great fear of downward motion.

Bryonia. Pain and pressure in stomach, sensitive to touch; nausea, vomiting; child is thirsty, wants to stay completely still and be left alone.

Carbolicum acidum. Seasickness with extreme nausea, vomiting, distention, terrible pains that come and go suddenly; sense of smell may be extremely acute.

Cocculus. Nausea, vertigo, headache, or sense of emptiness in the head; worse from smell of food; child talks quickly, yawns, feels numb; worse on getting cold.

Glonoine. Seasickness with dizziness, palpitation, pulsing sensation throughout the body; nausea and vomiting; worse from sun or heat.

Kali bichromium. Seasickness; vertigo and nausea from standing up; weakness; vomiting of bright yellow water.

Petroleum. Mouth waters excessively; child breaks out in cold sweat; headache in back of head and neck; empty, sick feeling in stomach, better from food, warmth.

Sepia. Nausea worse if child lies on her side; worse from sight or smell of food; dizziness; headache in forehead; child may crave sour things, be irritable.

Tabacum. Icy feet and hands, cold sweat, violent vomiting, terrible sinking feeling in the pit of the stomach, better in open air.

ACUPRESSURE AND MASSAGE. If the queasiness is not too serious, the child may rub these points himself while riding.

CV 12, 13: Tender points midway between the lower tip of the breastbone and the navel.

ST 36: A tender point next to the outer side of the big bump at the top of the shin.

P 6: A point in the mid-forearm, three of the child's finger-breadths above the palm-side wrist-crease.

- Gently rub the spot between the eyebrows.
- Rub the tender point right in the middle of the elbow crease.
- Find and rub all tender areas along the rim of the skull where it joins the neck.

MOUTH AND TONGUE

Clues to the state of a child's health can be found in the condition of the mouth, tongue, lips, breath, and teeth. The tongue may be coated during a cold or digestive upset. A sore mouth can be the result of nutritional deficiencies or infection, or of injuries to the mouth membranes or gums (such as accidentally biting the cheek or tongue, improper toothbrushing, or irritation from jagged teeth or braces). A tongue with a very red tip or sides may be a sign of emotional stress. Sores in the mouth may be caused by several kinds of infection.

Rarely, the cause of a mouth condition may be a foreign substance or chemical, or a serious condition such as gangrene or tumors.

SORES IN THE MOUTH

A tingling sensation in the lining of the mouth is often the forerunner of canker sores: small, inflamed white or yellow oval ulcers. The sores may make it hurt to talk or eat. They usually show up when the child is under nervous stress or tired and run-down, and usually last one to two weeks. Allergy to wheat or other foods may be a contributing cause. For treatment, see COLD SORES.

THRUSH (Candidiasis)

Thrush is a yeast infection in the mouth that is not uncommon in babies and children. White patches that look like cottage cheese curds show up on the membranes of the mouth or tongue, later turning to red or bleeding ulcers.

WHAT A PHYSICIAN MAY DO

A doctor will probably prescribe nystatin, an anti-yeast medication.

WHAT YOU CAN DO AT HOME

Poor nutrition, tiredness, or treatment with antibiotics or cortisone may predispose a child to thrush. Extra vitamins and minerals, and milk cultured with acidophilus (yogurt, kefir) should be given to help build up resistance to the yeast; or add powdered acidophilus from capsules or tablets to water and, several times a day, have the child rinse his mouth and swallow it. Make a brew of goldenseal and have the child use it as a rinse, several times a day.

HOMEOPATHIC REMEDIES.

Borax. A nursing baby may pull away from the nipple; mouth is dry and hurts; child may have strong fear of downward motion.

Mercurius vivus. Bad breath; sore mouth; drooling; sore or bleeding gums; puffy, coated tongue.

Sulphur. Mouth is sore, bright red, and burns (try if *Mercurius* doesn't work).

TRENCH MOUTH
This is an infection of the gums, mouth, and throat with painful, bleeding sores, drooling, and bad-smelling breath.

WHAT A PHYSICIAN MAY DO
Doctors or dentists may scrape away the diseased tissue and give antibiotics if the infection is thought to be associated with bacteria.

WHAT YOU CAN DO AT HOME
Raising the child's resistance through rest and good nutrition is the best remedy. Avoid all processed and refined foods. Give fresh fruit and vegetable juices, broths, soft foods; avoid acidic or spicy foods that may sting. Rinsing the mouth with salt water or a brew of goldenseal is helpful. Echinacea tea will help fight infection. Massaging the gums with powdered myrrh can help.

For herbs, homeopathic remedies, and acupressure points, see INFECTIONS.

DRY MOUTH
If mouth dryness occurs during fever, or follows any condition that causes fluids to be lost from the body (diarrhea, vomiting, excessive perspiration), it may mean the child is becoming dehydrated, especially if her eyes look sunken and her skin shows a loss of elasticity (see DEHYDRATION). Dry mouth or excessive thirst may be a sign of diabetes (see DIABETES). Dryness of the mouth may be a side effect or overdose effect of certain medications, such as antihistamines.

DIFFICULTY OPENING THE MOUTH
Slight dislocation of the jaw joint (TMJ) and disorders of the bite may be responsible for difficulty in opening the mouth. Jaw misalignments are often accompanied by neck and shoulder pain. Some practitioners, particularly cranially oriented chiropractors and certain dentists, can help correct such problems.

Difficulty opening the mouth is often due to inflammation, swelling, or muscle tightness during sore throat, mumps, or tooth or gum infection.

If the muscles of the jaw have grown very stiff, and the child has had a puncture wound (from a nail, thorn, animal bite, etc.) within the last few weeks, tetanus should be suspected. This is a very dangerous condition that needs a doctor's attention at once.

TONGUE CONDITIONS

When the tongue becomes red, sore, or swollen, the cause is usually an injury (a burn from hot food or drink, a cut from ice or a sharp object, a scrape from broken teeth) or irritation from foods, condiments, medicine, or chemicals. A sore tongue may also reflect a disorder somewhere else in the body, such as sluggish digestion, anemia, a nutritional deficiency, or liver or thyroid problems. A tongue with a very red tip and sides may be a sign of emotional stress.

A tongue that has been bitten or cut usually heals fairly quickly. Until it heals the diet should be limited to juices and broths that don't sting, and to soft, bland foods such as bananas, yogurt, and tofu. If the tongue is inflamed for other reasons, B vitamins, iron (preferably as ferrous gluconate), vitamins C and E may be helpful.

The tongue may become coated white or yellow during an illness or digestive troubles. Some people recommend brushing the tongue at the same time as brushing the teeth; not all children can do this without gagging. Fortunately, if the child is healthy and well nourished there is often no need to do it at all.

Mumps

Mumps is a viral infection, the main symptom of which is swollen salivary glands. The largest salivary gland—the parotid—is found in the cheek, in front of and below the ear. This gland may enlarge on one or both sides, and dramatically change the shape of the face. Swelling can start on one side and later come up on the other. If the edge of the child's jawbone can't be felt below the ear, his earlobe seems pushed out by swelling, or he feels an intense stinging pain inside his cheek when trying to eat sour fruit, pickles, salad dressings, or spicy foods, he may have mumps. Fever, headache, and either dry mouth or excessive salivation may be other symptoms. Some cases are so mild they are hardly noticed.

Mumps begin to be contagious two days before the symptoms appear. After exposure, two to three weeks may pass before the illness shows up. Some parents may choose to expose a small child to mumps on purpose, since cases are much milder in small children; in teenagers and adults, the testicles, ovaries, pancreas, thyroid, heart, or nervous system may become involved. A case of the mumps usually lasts from seven to ten days, and is likely to give lifetime immunity. Vaccinations are much less efficient and should usually be avoided.

Signs of complications may be: swelling of the testicles, ovaries, or breasts; impaired hearing; abdominal pain and vomiting (which may be signs of pancreatitis); intense headache, very stiff neck, abnormal lethargy, dizziness, spots of bleeding under the skin or delirium (see MENINGITIS). If a child has any of these symptoms, see a doctor immediately.

WHAT A PHYSICIAN MAY DO

Doctors often recommend aspirin or acetaminophen to help reduce pain or fever in mumps; these should not be used since they may interfere with the body's disease-fighting processes and often have serious side effects.

If there are complications, keep in close touch with a doctor and watch for signs of emergency. For swollen testicles, doctors may recommend home care measures such as ice packs and rest. Mumps-related pancreatitis usually goes away within a week or so; if lots of fluids are lost through vomiting, they may be replaced intravenously. If encephalitis or meningitis occurs, the child will be hospitalized and treated with antibiotics.

WHAT YOU CAN DO AT HOME

PRACTICAL MEASURES. Rest is a good idea, but there is usually no need for a small child to stay in bed. He should be kept away from teenagers and adults who have never had the mumps. Teenagers should rest in bed until all fever is gone.

If the swelling is very uncomfortable, a clean piece of flannel wrapped around the throat and neck often feels good. Applying cool damp cloths, a poultice of mullein herb in damp cotton cloth, or a banana-skin poultice may be soothing.

NUTRITION. Give nonacidic fluids and soft foods (such as pureed fruit, broths and soups, tofu); avoid sour, strong, or spicy foods that may hurt or sting. For vitamins, see INFECTIONS.

HERB TEAS. Echinacea, red clover; cloves (two to a cup) simmered in apple juice.

HOMEOPATHIC REMEDIES.

Aconitum napellus. Sudden fever, agitation, thirst; worse with warmth and better in fresh air.

Apis mellifica. Swelling is very tender, puffy, and pink; lack of thirst.

Arsenicum album. Exhausted and anxious, chilly, thirsty for sips; worse after midnight; testicles, ovaries, or other body parts may be swollen.

Belladonna. High fever, flushed skin, shooting pain, throbbing headache; right side may be most swollen; child is very restless, sensitive to light, may be delirious.

Bryonia. Hard, tender swelling; any motion hurts; child is grumpy, has a dry mouth, is very thirsty; swelling may disappear abruptly but child seems worse.

Carbo vegetabilis. Slow fever; pale or bluish skin; indigestion; child craves air and is chilly; testicles, ovaries, other parts of the body may be involved.

Mercurius vivus. Salivary glands hard and painful, those under chin may also be swollen; child has bad breath, excessive saliva; sweating, especially at night.

Pulsatilla. Symptoms last a long time; may involve ovaries, breasts, testicles; child is weepy, thirstless, worse with warmth and at night; better in fresh air.

Rhus toxicodendron. Dark red swelling, may be more on the left side; child feels achy, better from moving around. (This may help prevent mumps in adults who have been exposed.)

For acupressure and massage, see FEVER and INFECTIONS.

MUSCLE CRAMPS

A cramp is a sudden, painful, involuntary contraction of a muscle. Cramps are usually felt in legs, fingers, neck, and back, or in the muscle tissue of internal organs such as the uterus or intestines. Cramps can be caused by extra stress and fatigue, poor digestion and assimilation of nutrients, dietary deficiencies, loss of body salt, overexertion, shoes with poor arch support, allergy, hormonal shifts, or may accompany certain diseases such as colds and flu. Cramps may also occur near broken bones or be symptoms of disorders such as diabetes, hepatitis, polio, and tetanus.

WHAT A PHYSICIAN MAY DO

A thorough physical examination may be given to screen for serious diseases. Some physicians will assess diet, salt balance, exercise, and overall health habits. Some prescribe muscle relaxants. These drugs only alter symptoms; they do not correct the cause of the cramps. They also have very dangerous side effects.

WHAT YOU CAN DO AT HOME

PRACTICAL MEASURES. If a child wakes in the night with painful leg cramps, get her to take repeated, quick, short panting breaths (similar to the breathing used in some techniques of natural childbirth); this can reduce the sensation of pain.

Massage and heat (warm applications or a soak in the tub) are helpful unless there is a new injury in the area of cramping, in which case heat will make swelling and inflammation worse.

Poultices of comfrey root or raspberry leaves may ease a cramping muscle.

NUTRITION. Fresh fruits and vegetables, especially carrots, beets, cucumbers, and alfalfa sprouts, should be eaten every day. Extra calcium, magnesium, B-complex, and adequate vitamin E will help.

HERB TEAS. Chamomile, dandelion root, raspberry leaf, parsley, peppermint, alfalfa.

ACUPRESSURE AND MASSAGE.
> LV 14: A tender point on the front of the rib cage, midway between the nipple and the lower ribs.
> LV 3: A tender point midway between the first and second metatarsal bones.
> KI 1: A point on the side between the pads of the ball of the foot.
> KI 3: The tender point just behind the upper rear aspect of the inner anklebone.

NAUSEA AND VOMITING

A child may feel nauseous—sick and queasy—for a great number of reasons, among them excitement, nervousness, motion sickness, overeating, allergy, and infection. Other causes may be ingestion of unwholesome foods, nonfood substances (such as dirt, starch, modeling clay) or swallowed mucus during colds. Poisons and medications can also cause nausea. Nausea is often followed by vomiting, one of the body's unpleasant but effective methods of clearing out unwanted substances. Children have sensitive stomachs and may vomit more easily than adults; they seem less capable of holding it back, so they often "get it over with" and feel better more quickly.

If the vomit has flecks of blood in it and the child is not feverish, the force of vomiting may have slightly injured the membranes of the esophagus. Blood in vomit may also have come from a very recent nosebleed. If a child has frequent nausea and stomach pain, these may be signs that an ulcer is forming. If there is blood in the stool and intense abdominal pain along with vomiting, a doctor should examine the child right away.

A child should see a doctor if vomiting is severe and can't be controlled, if he is not able to keep small sips of fluid down, if he has high fever, is delirious, or has other signs of serious illness. Migraine headaches, head injuries, hepatitis, pancreatic problems, urinary tract infections, meningitis, aneurysms, and tumors may bring on nausea or vomiting, but most of these are rare. (See specific sections; also FEVER and DEHYDRATION.)

WHAT A PHYSICIAN MAY DO

If a child has become dehydrated from vomiting, intravenous fluids may be given along with electrolytes to restore the chemical balance in the blood. Drugs that prevent vomiting (usually antihistamines, as pill or suppository) are sometimes prescribed. Such medications should be given only in extreme and well-understood cases; they can cause serious disturbances in the child's system.

WHAT YOU CAN DO AT HOME

PRACTICAL MEASURES AND NUTRITION. Don't give the child anything she can't keep down. Even if the vomiting has done its job and removed the unwanted material, the digestive tract may need time to calm itself.

To restore lost fluids, give small amounts of water, juice, teas, or broth every few minutes, or let the child suck on ice chips or frozen fruit juice bars; do this in very small doses, gradually; slow down if too much fluid brings more vomiting. When the child has kept fluids down for several hours and is ready to eat, start with something light that she likes, like crackers, dry toast, light soups, or applesauce. (See also INDIGESTION AND GAS, FLU, MOTION SICKNESS and the Poisoning section in Part Two.)

HERB TEAS. Peppermint, spearmint, raspberry leaf, slippery elm, chamomile.

HOMEOPATHIC REMEDIES. (See also INDIGESTION AND GAS, MOTION SICKNESS.)

Aconitum napellus. Nausea and vomiting with fever, thirst, sweat; everything but water may taste bitter; child is very anxious or frightened.

Antimonium crudum. Burps taste of food; vomiting after overeating or eating nonfood substances; tongue coated white; child dislikes being touched or looked at.

Arsenicum album. Violent vomiting, exhaustion, burning or cramping pain, chilliness; thirsty, but drinks in small sips; worse after midnight; child feels sicker from the smell or thought of food; from spoiled food, too much fruit, food poisoning.

Bryonia. Child wants to lie perfectly still; slight motions may bring on vomiting; dry mouth, thirst, but vomits right after drinking; nausea from fatty food.

Chamomilla. Nausea, sweat after eating or drinking; stomach acid rises, bitter taste; vomiting; cramping pain in stomach; child may be flushed, irritable, angry.

Colocynthis. Intense, cramping pains better from hard pressure or bending double; vomiting; bitter taste; tongue may feel rough or scalded; after indignation.

Ipecacuanha. Violent vomiting, nausea remaining afterward; lots of mucus and salivation; vomiting triggered by coughing; child does not always feel horribly ill.

Nux vomica. Sour taste, nausea; stomach pain; worse in morning and from eating; retching, feels urge to vomit but can't; child is irritable, pushy.

Phosphorus. Burning pain, nausea, feeling of emptiness and nagging hunger; vomiting after warm drinks; thirst; cold water relieves nausea, but is vomited once it has warmed in stomach; child may feel weak, fearful, likes ice cream.

Pulsatilla. Nausea from rich food, overeating; food may be vomited up after many hours, only partly digested; tongue coated thick white or yellow; child may be weepy and clinging; worse at night or in a stuffy room.

Veratrum album. Violent vomiting alternating with diarrhea; thirst; cramping in arms and legs; child is weak and very chilly.

ACUPRESSURE AND MASSAGE.

LI 4: The point at the end of the crease between the thumb and index finger.

CV 12, 13: Tender points midway between the lower tip of the breastbone and the navel.

P 6: A point in the mid-forearm, three of the child's finger-breadths above the palm-size wrist-crease.

ST 36: A tender point next to the outer side of the big bump at the top of the shin.

GB 40: A tender point just below the lower front aspect of the outer anklebone.

LV 3: A tender point midway between the first and second metatarsal bones.

NOSE CONDITIONS

The nose draws in, cleans, and warms the air we breathe and sends information to the parts of the brain that decode and interpret smells. The most common problems children experience with their noses are bumps and bruises, symptoms of colds and allergies, and nosebleeds.

INJURIES

When a nose gets bumped—by a swinging door, a brother's head, or a soccer ball—it can swell so much that the contours of bone and cartilage can't be seen sufficiently to tell if it is broken. Any bleeding should be controlled (see below). If the nose is not bleeding, put ice in a clean, damp cloth and apply it right away to slow the swelling. After a few days, the swelling will go down enough to reveal the nose's shape. If it is bent or altered, a doctor will give a local anesthetic and realign it. If, at any time, the pain is extreme, the nose is distinctly crooked, or breathing is blocked on one side, see a doctor right away.

RHINITIS

This is when the mucous membranes of the nose are inflamed and swollen, making it stuffed up or runny. Rhinitis is usually part of a viral infection or allergy, but can be caused by a foreign object. (See COLDS, ALLERGIES, FOREIGN OBJECTS.)

NOSEBLEED (Epistaxis)

Most of children's bloody noses are mild and stop bleeding within an hour. Bleeding usually comes from tiny capillaries in the lower middle of the fleshy front part of the nose. Even if it seems profuse it is rarely serious. These small blood vessels can be injured when the lining of the nose has become irritated, as from dry indoor air, a cold, allergy, injury, vigorous nose-blowing, or nose-picking.

If bleeding is profuse and doesn't slow down significantly within half an hour, or if the child has very frequent nosebleeds that have no apparent cause, call a doctor. If the nosebleed is caused by a fall or forceful head injury—especially if the child shows other symptoms such as drowsiness, disorientation, vomiting, or unconsciousness—it is essential to have a physician check him right away.

WHAT A PHYSICIAN MAY DO

A doctor will examine the nose to try to pinpoint the source of the bleeding. Sometimes a pledget of cotton, soaked with a solution that constricts the blood vessels, is placed in the nostril. Silver nitrate applied to the blood vessel or electrocautery may be used to seal off a broken vessel. The doctor may check for growths in the nose, signs of dietary deficiency, infection, or disease. He may check the child's blood pressure. If it is high, attempts will be made to lower it through change of diet and habits or with medication.

WHAT YOU CAN DO AT HOME

PRACTICAL MEASURES. If the bleeding doesn't stop by itself within a minute or two, have the child—sitting up—blow his nose to remove any mucus that might keep a clot from forming; then pinch his nostrils together (including most of the front half of the nose) while he breathes though his mouth. Doing this is usually enough to stop a nosebleed in five to twenty minutes. Don't stop to check too early or too frequently, or you might interrupt the clotting. After the bleeding stops, don't let him touch the clot for at least an hour, even if it bothers him.

Putting the child's feet in ice or cold water, or putting an ice pack on the back of his neck, may sometimes slow the bleeding.

To prevent nosebleeds caused by dry indoor air (often a result of electric or woodburning heat), the air should be humidified by using a vaporizer, turning on the shower periodically, or keeping a pot of water boiling on the stove.

Nose-picking should be discouraged. If the child picks his nose because of itching or irritation, a little oil or vaseline on the walls of the nostrils may help.

Any allergies (to pollen, animal dander, dust, tobacco smoke, feathers, mattress stuffing, etc.) that may be causing irritation or congestion should be tracked down. Frequent nosebleeds are sometimes related to milk allergy.

NUTRITION. Foods such as citrus fruits, bell peppers, alfalfa sprouts, and other fresh fruits and vegetables high in vitamin C and bioflavonoids can help prevent nosebleeds. Supplements of bioflavonoids and vitamins C, E, and A may help.

HERB TEAS. Rose hip, comfrey, lemon peel, nettle, shepherd's purse.

HOMEOPATHIC REMEDIES.
    Arnica montana. Any nosebleed, especially one from injury.
    Ipecacuanha. Profuse, spurting bleeding.
    Phosphorus. Heavy or frequent bleeding that starts while blowing the nose.

ACUPRESSURE AND MASSAGE.
- Pinch the center of the margin of the thumb-webs on both hands.
- Pull the first middle-finger knuckle on the same side as the bleeding nostril.
- Hold the arm on the same side as the bleeding nostril up in the air.

PNEUMONIA

Pneumonia is, technically, the presence of fluid in the lungs. This occurs when the lungs' deeper air sacs (called alveoli) become inflamed. Sometimes this inflammation is minor and short-term; sometimes it is very serious. Although pneumonia occurs in differing degrees of severity, it always requires a doctor's attention. It is sometimes seen in children as a complication of chicken pox, measles, or neglected colds.

There are two basic kinds of pneumonia. Bacterial pneumonia is more serious and has more violent symptoms. The child may come down suddenly with shuddering chills followed by high fever, prostration or delirium, and a deep, painful cough that may bring up bloody or rust-colored phlegm. The breathing can be very rapid, and the child sweaty and fearful. The child may also have headache, nausea, vomiting, or convulsions. These symptoms are difficult to mistake. If they occur, medical help should be found right away.

Children who feel run-down, with mild fever and chills, a bad cough bringing up normal-colored mucus, and fluid sounds in their lungs often have a condition diagnosed as atypical, virus, or walking pneumonia.

WHAT A PHYSICIAN MAY DO

The doctor will give the child a general examination, and listen to the chest to assess the type and location of breathing sounds heard (or not heard). Many doctors take X rays, looking for evidence of fluid in the lungs; this is rarely necessary, since nothing may show up on the films even if pneumonia is present—or indications of pneumonia may show on X ray even when the case is not serious. X ray findings therefore make no significant difference in treatment; the child should be spared the radiation.

A culture of sputum (the stuff coughed up) will usually tell which bacteria (if any) are involved in the infection, and an antibiotic will probably be prescribed. "Walking" or "viral" pneumonia is often associated with the mycoplasma organism, which is not really a virus; mycoplasma may be affected by the antibiotics tetracycline and erythromycin, and these are sometimes prescribed for children when walking pneumonia is diagnosed. Antibiotics should be used only when pneumonia is bacterial, or serious; some doctors prescribe penicillin or other antibiotics for viral pneumonia to prevent further complications, even though bed rest and good nutrition will usually bring the child back to health just as quickly (within a few days to weeks). If you know or suspect that your child has an allergy to *any* drug, be sure to tell the doctor so a bad reaction does not ensue.

In serious cases, in very small children, or in cases with signs of dehydration, observation and supportive hospital care (with fluid and salt replacement, oxygen tent or breathing tube) will be advised. If a hospital stay is necessary, make sure that someone familiar to the child is always there, so she will not be frightened or lonely.

Some doctors will administer high doses of vitamin C intravenously along with (or in place of) antibiotics. Vitamin C can support the child's immune function and protect against the toxic effects of drugs. Parents have a right to insist on this sort of treatment—but whether it is provided depends on the habits and orientation of the doctor and hospital. If possible, look for open-minded doctors, and prepare ahead of time.

WHAT YOU CAN DO AT HOME

PRACTICAL MEASURES. Nutritional, herbal, or homeopathic remedies may be begun right away and are often effective. If the symptoms continue to be severe, however, use standard medical treatment as well.

Have the child wear cotton pajamas and lie in bed between cotton or flannel sheets. A hot-water bottle or heating pad on her feet or stomach may give some relief. Rubbing a "tea" of gray lichen from oak trees (one teaspoonful simmered in a cup of water) on the chest, or a compress of ginger or oil of cloves, can help ease discomfort.

NUTRITON. A liquid diet of broths, citrus juices, and grape juice may help conserve energy for recovery. (See also COUGH.) Extra vitamin A, very high doses of C, and balanced B-complex (with extra B_6) are useful.

HERB TEAS. Echinacea, ginger, coltsfoot, horehound, wild cherry bark.

HOMEOPATHIC REMEDIES. (See also COUGH and FEVER.)

Aconitum napellus. Sudden onset; child has rapid, hard pulse, hot skin, violent symptoms, thirst with great anxiety. (This is often needed at the beginning of an illness.)

Antimonium tartaricum. Feels very weak, coughs up frothy mucus, has great oppression of the chest, and may feel like vomiting. (This is an especially useful remedy for infants.)

Bryonia. Wants to lie still, putting pressure on the side that hurts; he feels stitches in his chest from breathing, and pain with even slight movement; he coughs up tough, rust-colored mucus, feels dry-mouthed, thirsty, constipated.

Phosphorus. Tight chest and painful cough, worse lying on the left side; coughs up greenish or yellowish phlegm that may be streaked with blood; breath sounds like crackling or sawing; pulse is very rapid; may remain alert even with very high fever; thirsty for ice-cold drinks, although drinking, talking, and laughing may bring on more coughing.

ACUPRESSURE AND MASSAGE.

LU 1: A tender point in the indentation below the shoulder end of the collarbone.

LI 11: A tender point at the thumb-side end of the elbow-crease when the arm is bent.

LI 4: The point at the end of the crease between the thumb and index finger.

ST 36: A tender point next to the outer side of the big bump at the top of the shin.

SP 6: A tender point three of the child's finger-breadths above the inner anklebone.

POISON OAK, IVY, AND SUMAC

These plants grow in many areas of brush and woodland. They contain a toxic oil that can come into contact with skin and tissues, and cause a bumpy, streaky, blistery, itching rash. Contact can occur by walking past and brushing against the leaves, twigs, or berries themselves—or by touching an animal, rug, towel, toy, tool, piece of clothing, or other object that has somehow picked up some oil. Smoke from burning the plants can also carry oil to skin, eyes, mouth, and breathing passages. The irritation and inflammation appear from hours to days after exposure and last from days to weeks. The rash can't be spread by scratching, but in the early stage—before the outbreak—the oil can be spread by rubbing the face and eyes or touching other body parts. Because sensitivity to the oil is an allergy, outbreaks can increase in intensity with each exposure; some people think they are not sensitive, and later receive a distressing surprise. Extreme cases may need a physician's treatment, even a hospital stay.

WHAT A PHYSICIAN MAY DO

Doctors may recommend over-the-counter remedies such as calamine lotion or aluminum acetate (Burow's solution) for mild cases, and prescribe cortisone for severe ones. Cortisone can have adverse effects on many body processes. It is better to use natural remedies that soothe skin eruptions rather than chemicals that suppress them. Some calamine lotions also contain an anesthetic to which some children are allergic; this can make the rash and itching worse.

WHAT YOU CAN DO AT HOME

PRACTICAL MEASURES. Show the plants to your child so he knows what they look like in all seasons and can stay away from them. Have him wear long pants and socks when he is walking through places in which these plants grow.

If you think anyone has touched the plant, immediately use soap and warm water to wash all parts of the skin that could possibly have been exposed, then wash again in several hours. All clothes and objects that could have oil on them should be thoroughly cleaned.

Scratching should be discouraged so the rash does not become infected.

Warm baths may soothe the itching, with oatmeal (one cup to a tub of water); baking soda (one-half cup to a tub); or sage tea (four ounces of herb simmered in a quart of water and strained) added to the bathwater. Take care to keep the temperature comfortable. After the bath, have the child stand in a warm place and dry in the air.

Poultices of crushed plantain leaves, wheat bran, clay, and goldenseal may help relieve the itching. Apply calendula tincture (diluted 5:1), cooled sage tea, aloe vera gel, comfrey root, and slippery-elm powders, vitamin E oil, lemon juice, or a paste of baking soda and water to the rash.

NUTRITION. The child should consume plenty of fresh fruit and vegetable juices, especially carrot juice. All refined, processed, fried, or very spicy foods should be avoided. Extra vitamin C, B-complex with pantothenic acid, calcium and magnesium supplements will help reduce the rash and itching.

HOMEOPATHIC REMEDIES.
Anacardium orientale. Big blisters filled with fluid; rash may be worse on the face; itch made worse by hot applications.
Belladonna. Rash hot, bright red, and throbbing; child may be restless, feverish.
Bryonia. Dry, bumpy rash; child irritable, does not want to move or be disturbed.
Graphites. Eruptions ooze sticky golden fluid; itch worse at night and from warmth.
Ledum palustre. Rash puffy, itching; worse from warmth; relieved by cold applications.
Rhus toxicodendron. Burning, intense itching, blisters; worse at night and from scratching; relief from very hot water; child is restless, anxious, feels better moving around.
Sepia. Dry, scaly brown or reddish rash; child feels better being warm, but itch is worse from the warmth of the bed or sweating.
Sulphur. Very red, irritated, itchy skin, worse from scratching and washing; child may feel hot and sensitive to heat.

PUNCTURE WOUNDS

Children's puncture wounds are most often incurred by stepping on tacks, exposed nails, or thorns, or by poking fingers with needles or sharp objects. Since such wounds are often small on the surface but deep, they can be hard to clean out, and it may be difficult for air to reach the injured tissues for proper healing.

This is dangerous because tetanus (often a fatal disease) requires just such airless conditions to develop. The bacteria responsible for tetanus may be found in any kind of dirt, particularly soil containing animal excrement; the microorganisms themselves do not cause the disease, but—in a closed and airless environment—they may proliferate and produce a nerve toxin that can cause distressing, life-threatening symptoms.

Call a doctor right away if: the punctured skin was very dirty; the sharp object went through a shoe; an object has broken off in a wound; the wound was made by glass which may not have all come out; or the wound seems red, hot, swollen, tender, or otherwise infected.

WHAT A PHYSICIAN MAY DO

The doctor will open and clean the wound and check for the presence of foreign objects; this may require probing or cutting. Sometimes an X ray is made if the object is thought to be metal. The doctor will want to give a tetanus shot if the child's immunizations are not "up to date." (See Immunizations in Part Two.) Antibiotics, in ointment or pill form, may be prescribed to prevent infection.

WHAT YOU CAN DO AT HOME

PRACTICAL MEASURES. Try to make the wound bleed by gently pressing the tissues around it; bleeding will help carry out the dirt and bacteria. If it is already bleeding, don't try to stop it unless the blood is spurting out. (If blood is spurting from the wound, but you think a foreign object may still be in it, do not stop the bleeding by pressing *on* the wound; move slightly closer to the heart and apply pressure there. Call 911 or go to an emergency room immediately.)

Unless it is trivial, the wound should be gently opened as much as possible and thoroughly cleaned with soap and water or hydrogen peroxide. Soak the injured part in warm water for half an hour several times a day to keep it clean and open, as well as to increase the circulation to speed healing.

Ledum tincture or Hypericum tincture may be applied directly to the wound several times a day, or put in the soaking-water. A poultice made of tobacco mixed with water to form a paste, left on twenty-four hours, may help prevent tetanus, if no other help is available.

Homeopathic Remedies.

Ledum palustre Any puncture wound, especially if it is red, swollen, throbbing, and feels cold to the touch but pain is relieved by cold applications.

Hypericum. Sharp, shooting pains; especially if the injury is in the toes or fingertips.

Apis mellifica. Wound is quite swollen and pink, stings, and feels hot.

For other natural remedies, see CUTS AND SCRAPES and INFECTIONS.

RABIES

Rabies is an extremely serious viral disease transmitted through the saliva of infected domestic or wild animals, particularly skunks, raccoons, squirrels, foxes, and bats. Rabid animals usually act strangely, often attack without being provoked, and sometimes foam at the mouth—but it is possible for a normal-seeming animal (especially a bat) to be a carrier.

Symptoms may appear a week after the bite, although forty days is the average incubation time; in some cases, symptoms do not show up until a year has passed. In humans, the symptoms of rabies infection include: persistent redness and inflammation at the site of the bite, even though the wound was healed; irritability or depression, followed eventually by wildness or excitability; drooling caused by an inability to swallow because of muscle spasms in the throat; the person may become so thirsty that the sight of water brings on horrible agitation—hence the other name for rabies, hydrophobia; paralysis, usually appearing within three to ten days of the earliest symptoms, followed by coma, asphyxia, and death.

WHAT A PHYSICIAN MAY DO

The wound must be deeply cleaned and disinfected, and rabies antiserum may be injected into the wound. Rabies vaccine will then be given, in fourteen to twenty-one daily injections; after the initial series of shots is finished, boosters are given on the tenth and twentieth days.

If it is likely that a child was exposed to rabies through an animal bite, it is important that she receive the treatment, because the untreated disease is invariably fatal.

WHAT YOU CAN DO AT HOME

PRACTICAL MEASURES. If possible, locate the animal that bit the child, but do not get near it. If the animal seems ill, foams at the mouth, or acts strangely—frenzied, belligerent, or even uncommonly friendly—take the bitten child to a doctor or emergency room right away. If the owner can't be found or the animal is wild, call an animal-control agency or the police. The animal should be observed for signs of rabies (and confined if necessary) for fifteen days.

Clean the bite and treat it to prevent infection. (See BITES and PUNCTURE WOUNDS.) Extra vitamins C, E, A, and zinc should be given to help immune function.

Daily "Turkish baths" or steam baths in which the room is very warm and the air filled with vapor have been reported in older medical books (written before the rabies antiserum was developed) to be successful in treatment of rabies.

HOMEOPATHIC REMEDIES. For help with the child's general state of health, consult an experienced homeopathic practitioner. *Cantharis* has been cited in older books as a preventative for rabies. *Hydrophobinum* (a nosode) has also been used. *Belladonna, Hyoscyamus,* and *Stramonium* have been reported useful if the illness has advanced to the hydrophobic and convulsive states.

ACUPRESSURE AND MASSAGE.
>LI 4: The point at the end of the crease between the thumb and index finger.
>LI 11: A tender point at the thumb-side end of the elbow-crease when the arm is bent.
>LV 3: A tender point midway between the first and second metatarsal bones.
>ST 36: A tender point next to the outer side of the big bump at the top of the shin.
>SP 6: A tender point three of the child's finger-breadths above the inner anklebone.

CAUTION: The above natural measures and remedies are *not sub-stitutes* for immediate medical attention, and are not mentioned here as cures for rabies, although they may be useful as adjunctive therapy.

ROSEOLA

When a baby between six months and three years of age has a very high fever for several days (seventy-two hours is average), with no sign of earache, cough, abdominal pain, difficulty when urinating, or other explanation, he probably has roseola. Roseola is often the first dramatic disease a child has. The fever may reach 105 degrees F. Aside from nontender swollen lymph nodes behind the ears and at the back of the skull, and maybe a slight runny nose or red throat, this fever is the only symptom until the third or fourth day. The fever then drops, and a pink, patchy rash appears, mostly on the trunk. The rash usually lasts about twenty-four hours.

Roseola is contagious; the cause is not known but is thought to be a virus. If you know your child has been exposed, look for the fever in about one to two weeks. Because the fever is so high and rises so rapidly, the child may have a convulsion (see CONVULSIONS). It is hard for parents not to worry when there is such a high, unexplained fever, but complications from roseola are very rare.

If you are fairly sure your child has roseola, there is no need to see a doctor. If you are not sure, the doctor can examine the child to rule out other causes of fever. If the rash lasts for more than three days or becomes dark-colored, or if the child feels quite uncomfortable, pulls at her ears, or has a tummyache, check with a doctor.

WHAT A PHYSICIAN MAY DO
Doctors will usually prescribe acetaminophen or aspirin to bring down the fever.

WHAT YOU CAN DO AT HOME
PRACTICAL MEASURES. A fever is no fun, and—especially if this is his first one—the child will need a lot of extra attention and com-

forting. Try to reduce the temperature a little by sponging him with tepid water or peppermint tea and giving him cool drinks.

For other natural measures, herb teas, homeopathic remedies, and acupressure points, see FEVER.

RUBELLA
(German Measles, Three-Day Measles)

Rubella is a mild disease in children, causing low-grade fever, slight headache, runny nose, swollen lymph nodes behind the ears and on the back of the skull and neck, and a rash of tiny red spots starting on the face and spreading to other parts of the body. It lasts, as its nickname implies, about three days. Sometimes the muscles ache a bit or joints feel a little stiff, but rubella is hardly ever uncomfortable, and many children who have it go about their business as usual.

The most drastic effect of rubella is on pregnant women and their developing babies. If a woman catches rubella within the first three months of pregnancy, her baby may be born with very serious birth defects—among them deafness, cataracts, mental retardation, heart deformities, and cleft palate. Because of this danger, a child with rubella should be kept away from any girls and women who might possibly be pregnant. Girls under child-bearing age, or older girls and women who are *sure* they are not pregnant, should probably make an effort to be exposed, however, because one case of rubella gives lifelong immunity, unlike the vaccination. (See Immunizations in Part Two.)

WHAT A PHYSICIAN MAY DO
A doctor's help is hardly ever needed in rubella, unless a girl or woman in her first three months of pregnancy has been exposed. In such a case, the doctor may give a gamma globulin injection in the hope of staving off the disease.

WHAT YOU CAN DO AT HOME
For practical measures, nutrition, herb teas, and acupressure, see FEVER.

HOMEOPATHIC REMEDIES.

> *Aconitum napellus.* Sudden onset, agitation, flushing, fever.
> *Belladonna.* Skin is hot and red; throbbing headache, fever, restlessness.
> *Ferrum phosphoricum.* Gradual onset, rosy cheeks, fever, chills, sweat, soft rapid pulse.
> *Pulsatilla.* Child is weepy and irritable, wants attention, feels better in fresh air.

If a girl or woman has been exposed to rubella and is or may be pregnant, some homeopathic practitioners may give a rubella nosode to help protect against infection and subsequent birth defects. The effectiveness of a nosode for treatment or prevention of this disease is not completely documented, but since this treatment is not dangerous, some patients may want to consider it. Consult an experienced homeopathic physician.

SCARLET FEVER

Scarlet fever was once an extremely dangerous disease, but most cases that have occurred over the last fifty years or so have been fairly mild. It is, basically, a case of strep throat accompanied by a rash. It begins with fever, chills, and sometimes nausea and vomiting. The pink-red rash comes out in tiny dots, especially on the face, chest, abdomen, and groin, so that the skin looks flushed. The area around the mouth appears pale, and the tongue becomes red and bumpy, a condition known as strawberry tongue. These symptoms last for two or three weeks, after which time some skin may peel. Complications may be inner-ear involvement (which can lead to deafness), kidney infection, and rheumatic fever. If the child seems very ill or does not respond to natural remedies, it is wise to consult a doctor.

WHAT A PHYSICIAN MAY DO

Antibiotics (usually penicillin) or erythromycin could be prescribed to get rid of the strep bacteria, and in hopes of preventing complications.

WHAT YOU CAN DO AT HOME

PRACTICAL MEASURES. The child's diet should be mostly liquid to help her conserve strength for fighting off the infection. Give nourishing broths, fresh fruit and vegetable juices.

Some children like a massage with olive oil, or malt vinegar diluted 1:4 with warm water.

HERB TEAS. Peppermint, comfrey, dill, coltsfoot, echinacea.

HOMEOPATHIC REMEDIES. (See also INFECTIONS, THROAT INFLAMMATIONS, FEVER.)

Arsenicum album. Child feels exhausted but also restless; rash is rosy and may be scanty; ulcerated throat, with foul breath.
Belladonna. Rash looks smooth and red; child is thirsty, restless, even delirious; throat very red and swollen, so it hurts to swallow.
Pulsatilla. Child may be weepy and clinging; insomnia, jerking limbs, pain in hands and feet.
Sulphur. Sometimes given after other remedies (including antibiotics) if child takes a long time getting well.

SINUSITIS

Children's sinuses (air cavities in the skull) are not completely developed until past the age of three. After that, sinusitis—a viral or bacterial inflammation of the sinus linings—can occur. Pain may be felt on one or both sides of the face, above the eyebrows, behind the eyes, or in the cheekbones. Pressure and blockage may be due to swollen membranes from a cold or allergy, a deviated nasal septum, tooth problems, inhalation of fumes or drugs, or a foreign object in the nose. The child may have fever and chills, yellow-green mucus, loss of the sense of smell, and a stuffy or throbbing feeling in the face. The illness usually lasts two or three days, without leading to further complications. If it lasts longer, returns frequently, or if the tissues around the eyes are tender and swollen, take the child to a doctor.

WHAT A PHYSICIAN MAY DO

If the infection is making the child very ill and the sinuses are full of infected matter, a doctor may give antibiotics. Some doctors prescribe sprays that constrict the blood vessels in the nasal membranes. Although these can temporarily relieve the swelling, when use is discontinued the membranes may overreact and swell even more. If the sinuses remain blocked or inflamed, your child may be referred to a specialist who can drain them or remove the obstructions so they can drain themselves.

WHAT YOU CAN DO AT HOME

PRACTICAL MEASURES. To help prevent sinusitis, check for respiratory or food allergies and treat them. (See ALLERGIES.)

Use a humidifier or herbal vapor baths. (See COLDS.) Have the child breathe through a warm wet washcloth placed over his nose and mouth, or apply compresses of hot water or ginger tea over the painful areas; use these applications only if the child likes the way they feel.

Have the child drink lots of fluids to keep the secretions moist, so they can drain more easily.

NUTRITION. Remove all dairy products from the diet for several months—or altogether, if the child seems allergic to them. Eating garlic, onions, and horseradish may have some anti-infective effect and may open congested sinuses. Give lots of fresh fruit and vegetable juices, especially carrot juice.

Extra vitamins C, A, B-complex, calcium, magnesium, zinc, bioflavonoids, and beta carotene are beneficial.

HERB TEAS. Echinacea, rose hips, red clover, parsley, hops, chickweed, mullein.

HOMEOPATHIC REMEDIES. (See also COLDS and HEADACHES.)
Hepar sulphuris calcareum. Pain in the root of the nose; head feels bruised; yellow-greenish discharge; child is irritable, worse from cold and drafts.
Kali bichromium. Sinus ache is like a mask or in small, very painful spots; lots of tough, stringy yellow mucus.
Mercurius vivus. Thick greenish discharge, swelling in nose; child may have bad breath; sweating, drooling during sleep; worse at night and in damp weather.

Pulsatilla. Stuffy nose and head worse in a warm, closed room and better in open air; changing posture makes the head hurt; child weepy, not thirsty.

Silicea. Throbbing or tearing face pain, worse with cold and damp; warmth and pressure relieve the pain; child sweats, wants head covered; worse from exertion.

ACUPRESSURE AND MASSAGE.

LI 20: The tender points where the creases of the cheek meet the nose.

LI 4: The point at the end of the crease between the thumb and index finger.

LU 7: The tender point on the undersurface of the thumb-side forearm bone, two of the child's thumb-widths above the palm-side wrist-crease.

LV 3: A tender point midway between the first and second metatarsal bones.

· With the right thumb and middle finger, press against the back of the neck just below the skull while touching the two sides of the forehead with left thumb and index finger and gently rock the head (GB 20 and GB 14).

· Gently rub the cheekbones in a circular motion, then massage down the lines that extend from the wings of the nose toward the mouth.

· Find the groove in the muscles just behind the ear, and massage down the front of the neck muscles and across the top of the collarbone.

· Firmly pinch the skin between the eyebrows for several seconds.

· Massage the undersides of both big toes.

SKIN CONDITIONS

The skin in many ways reflects a person's state of health, both physical and emotional, by its color, texture, and luster. Because it is so visible, people often feel that the skin should be kept clear at all costs—that rashes or eruptions should be eradicated as quickly as possible. Since the skin is responsible for eliminating waste from the body, however, it is important to distinguish between removing a skin problem by suppressing it (treating the surface symptoms but driving the problem inside to another, deeper level) and removing it (restoring the system to balance and bringing about real healing).

General care of the skin requires adequate but not excessive cleanliness, fresh air, exercise, nonirritating clothing, and good nutrition. Nutrients that particularly contribute to the health of the skin, and can strengthen it against susceptibility to infection and disorders, are: vitamin A, zinc, beta carotene, vitamin C, balanced B-complex including pantothenic acid, essential fatty acids, good-quality protein (especially from fish or nonanimal sources), and plenty of pure water and fresh fruit and vegetable juices.

Following is a list of common skin conditions and home care suggestions.

BIRTHMARKS

Babies are sometimes born with dark pink, flat marks (known as stork bites) on the back of the neck and forehead. Other marks, usually dark blue, called Mongolian spots, are seen on the low back and are sometimes mistaken for bruises. Neither of these needs treatment, and both usually go away.

Flat, tan marks that may look like coffee stains of various sizes and shapes will probably not go away, but they often get lighter as a child grows, and cause no harm. An exception to this is freckling in the armpit region and brown patches that may be an indication of neurofibromatosis, a sometimes serious genetic disease.

Growing dark brown spots should be evaluated by a doctor. (See MOLES below.)

Dark red birthmarks (port-wine stains) are often found on the neck but may be anywhere. Some fade, some don't. Certain birthmarks may be raised, soft, and blue or red (strawberry marks). These are called hemangiomas because they involve blood vessel tissues. Many of these go away on their own within five years or so, but some remain; if they are located on the face or in an inconvenient or easily irritated spot, they may be removed by laser surgery.

MOLES

Moles can be present at birth or develop at any time; they are usually dark brown or black, and can be flat, raised, or hairy. If a mole is bothersome because it is on the face, or in an area in which irritation and infection are a risk because clothing or another part of the body rubs against it, the mole can be removed surgically.

Although it does not often happen, some moles become cancerous. If a mole begins to change—bleeds, becomes sore, itchy, or ulcerated, increases in size—or if the skin around it changes color, develops growths, or nearby lymph nodes swell, have a doctor look at it right away.

PRICKLY HEAT

This is an itchy rash of tiny, raised white or red dots, caused by plugged sweat glands. It shows up most often during hot, humid weather, usually from dressing too warmly, or from emotional stress. Newborn babies are likely to get prickly heat because their sweat glands are just learning to work.

Choose clothes that are light and allow the air to circulate. Cotton is best. Use several layers if there are variations in temperature or drafts.

Vitamin C has an antihistamine effect: a 100-mg tablet can be dissolved in pure water and given to the baby from a teaspoon or bottle. Skin-washes made of baking soda (one-half teaspoon in a cup of water) or vitamin B_6 (one tablet crushed and dissolved in water) may be applied. Lukewarm broths from cooking oats and barley can be added to the baby's bathwater. Do not use soap. Keep the room warm and let the child dry off in the air.

SUNBURN

Some children have skin that is extra-sensitive to sunlight. They need to be gradually habituated to intense sun, or protected against it with clothes and natural sunscreen lotions. Depending on the altitude and cloud conditions, the sun can be intense enough to burn even in colder weather and at times when it does not appear to be particularly bright.

If a burn is badly blistered, or covers a great deal of the body surface, or is very painful, a doctor should see the child. (See BURNS.)

WHAT A PHYSICIAN MAY DO

If the sunburn is not too serious, a doctor may recommend an over-the-counter sunburn cream or spray. Drugstores sell preparations containing benzocaine (an anesthetic) for reducing sunburn pain. These can slow recovery and sometimes irritate the skin. If the burn is serious, or signs of dehydration are present, the doctor will treat the child for these. (See BURNS and DEHYDRATION.)

WHAT YOU CAN DO AT HOME

PRACTICAL MEASURES. Avoid intense sun exposure, especially between the hours of 10:00 A.M. and 3:00 P.M. Prevent burning by having the child wear light cotton clothing that covers most of her skin, or by using a natural sunscreen lotion. Lotions containing PABA (a member of the B-complex) can help block the sun's burning rays. Try a little at a time; some children are allergic to these. There are also natural sunscreens made with other active ingredients. If a child's skin burns easily, have her go out in the sun at first for only fifteen or twenty minutes or less, working up to longer periods.

New babies should not be out in direct sunlight for more than five or ten minutes. Have them wear bonnets or sunhats, and always protect their eyes.

Don't plaster a sunburn with heavy grease; the skin feels cooler and heals faster when exposed to air. Aloe vera juice or gel is soothing when applied to burns, as is a light vitamin E cream. (Be careful: vitamin E applied directly from the capsule may sting, so try it on a small area first, or mix the oil with skin cream or lotion.)

Baths with baking soda (one-half cup), oatmeal, or broth from cooking oats or barley added to the water can be soothing. Cool compresses, or poultices of plantain or comfrey leaves (wrapped in a clean, damp cotton cloth) will help ease a burn.

NUTRITION. Any child out in the sun a lot should drink plenty of pure water and fresh juices. Supplementing the diet with balanced B-complex vitamins including PABA and vitamin E can reduce the likelihood of burning. These are also useful taken after burning, along with vitamin C, calcium, magnesium, zinc, beta carotene, and natural vitamin A.

FROSTBITE

Children are more susceptible to frostbite than are adults. When ears, cheeks, nose, toes, and fingertips are exposed to very cold temperatures, the skin begins to tingle and feel numb, then becomes dark red and swollen. Eventually, it may turn gray or dead white. If the frostbitten part is not thawed right away, its tissues may be permanently destroyed.

WHAT A PHYSICIAN MAY DO

A doctor will thaw the frostbitten part and stimulate circulation. If the tissue is damaged and gangrene is a possibility, an anti-coagulant drug may be given. If the part is too badly damaged, amputation may be necessary.

WHAT YOU CAN DO AT HOME

A frostbitten-finger or toe should be put immediately inside the child's own armpit (or someone else's) so that body heat can warm it quickly. No pressure other than this should be put on the injured part, including that of clothing. If warm water (102–107 degrees F.) is available, the frostbitten part can be immersed in it. *Hot* water should never be used, since the skin has lost its feeling and the heat may further damage it. Walking or moving around—anything that will warm the whole child—can help by increasing circulation. Warm drinks such as cider or herb teas (especially sage in moderate amounts) are helpful.

The homeopathic remedy *Ruta graveolens* sometimes relieves the after effects of frostbite. See a physician if frostbite does not improve right away.

OTHER SKIN CONDITIONS

Skin problems may accompany other conditions. See ACNE, BOILS, CUTS AND SCRAPES, and INFECTIONS. For loss of skin elasticity, see DEHYDRATION. For yellowness of skin and eyewhites, see JAUNDICE and HEPATITIS. For pallor, see ANEMIA and the section on Shock in Part Two. For a rash accompanied by or following fever, see CHICKEN POX, MEASLES, ROSEOLA, RUBELLA, and SCARLET FEVER.

SLEEP PROBLEMS

Different children need different amounts of sleep. Some infants sleep twenty hours a day, some only ten. Children under a year old usually need about eighteen hours. From age one to four, fifteen hours is average; from age four to eight, about ten or twelve; after age eight, about nine hours. Some children need naps until they're five, others give them up by age two. The child's mood and energy during the day, and the ease or difficulty he has in getting up in the morning, indicate whether his sleep is sufficient.

Most children find it hard to go to bed at bedtime because they are interested in playing and won't acknowledge that they are tired. Some resist going to bed and have insomnia because they feel lonely in their rooms or are afraid of the dark. Children may also find it hard to sleep when they are worried about something, or if some part of their body hurts. If the adults or older family members have company after the children's bedtime, small children may feel curious or left out. Nutritional deficiencies may make it hard for children to relax and fall asleep.

WHAT A PHYSICIAN MAY DO

Some doctors try to track down the cause of recurrent insomnia. Others may simply deal with the symptom by prescribing medications. Children should *not* be given sedatives; medications that cause drowsiness can have dangerous or even fatal side effects. Also, the sleep brought on by drugs is not true, healthy, restorative sleep.

Gentle spinal and cranial manipulations from a chiropractor, osteopath, or craniosacral therapist may help with serious sleep disorders.

WHAT YOU CAN DO AT HOME

PRACTICAL MEASURES. Try to encourage less rambunctious activities as bedtime draws near. Make sure the child gets some special attention (quiet conversation, a song or story) before being expected to sleep. If he is anxious about something (nightmares, school pressures, arguments), let him talk about it. Give him a nightlight if he wants one or leave a light on in the hall. If there is anything in the child's room that frightens him in the dark (clothes on a hook can look like a person, pieces of furniture might be monsters), turn on the light and let him see what it is, or change the arrangement so that it doesn't scare him. After you leave the room, let him talk or sing if he wants, to keep himself company.

Make sure the child's mattress is firm and not saggy or lumpy; check to see that his bed is big enough, and that he likes the size of his pillow and the way it feels. Be sure the temperature in the room is not too cold or hot and that he has enough fresh air.

Sleeping with a pillow or little cloth bag stuffed with herbs can be soothing. Use lavender, hops, rosemary, rose petals, thyme, or basil.

Daily exercise, sports, or strenuous play earlier in the day can help the child's nerves be calm at night. Hot baths before bed are often relaxing, but some children are made more energetic by them.

NUTRITION. Eating a heavy meal too close to bedtime may interfere with sleep, but some children fall asleep more easily if they have a little snack in the evening.

Sipping a cup of warm milk before bed can supply the amino acid tryptophan, which has a natural sedative effect. (Note: This is the natural food form of tryptophan. Recent batches of l-tryptophan sold in supplement form seem to have been contaminated. This does not mean that tryptophan is bad: it is an amino acid required by the body for proper function.)

A teaspoonful of honey or molasses (given before brushing the teeth) can have a tranquilizing effect; this may be stirred into warm milk, or given straight.

Extra calcium, magnesium, and balanced B-complex can help bring sleep.

HERB TEAS. Hops, lemon balm, chamomile, peppermint, rose hips, dill, fennel. (Don't give teas right before bedtime if the child is inclined to bedwetting.)

HOMEOPATHIC REMEDIES. If a child has frequent insomnia, seek guidance from an experienced prescriber.

Aconitum napellus. Child is frightened, excitable, feverish, agitated, thirsty.

Belladonna. Child wants to sleep but can't, imagines or thinks he sees scary things; throbbing pulse, nightmares.

Chamomilla. Child is very irritable; insomnia from indigestion or abdominal pain.

Cocculus. Bad effects from lack of sleep; dizziness.

Coffea. Child can't sleep because of excitement (usually something pleasant).

Ignatia. Sleeplessness from sadness, grief, or distressing events.
Nux vomica. Child is nervous, irritable; sensitive to noise; sleepless from staying up too late; may wake up at dawn and not be able to fall back to sleep.
Pulsatilla. After rich foods or overeating; child dislikes a warm or stuffy room.
Silicea. Frequent nightmares, sleepwalking; child may feel chilly.
Sulphur. Child's feet heat up in bed and he sticks them out of the covers; itching skin; nightmares; child may wake up early, unable to go back to sleep.

ACUPRESSURE AND MASSAGE.
· Gentle back- and neckrubs or foot massage can be restful and comforting.
  HT 7: A point just below the wrist-crease on the little-finger side.
  SP 6: A tender point three of the child's finger-breadths above the inner anklebone.
  LV 3: A tender point midway between the first and second metatarsal bones.
· Hold the tender point just behind the mastoid (the bony bump behind the earlobe).
· Press the center of the bottoms of the heels for several minutes.
· Press against the index finger side of the large knuckle where the middle finger joins the hand. (The child may lie on her back or side and fall asleep while pressing one thumb against this point on the other hand.)

SPRAINS AND STRAINS

Children's bodies are, in general, more flexible than adults', so sprains and strains are less frequent for them, but an awkward twist or fall may cause an injury that needs special attention. Ankles, knees, wrists, and shoulders are common spots for sprains and strains.

Sprains occur when ligaments (the connective tissues that bind bones together) are stretched or partly torn. To check for this, have the child hold still while you move the injured part. The injury is a sprain if pain is felt on this kind of passive movement. Damaged ligaments may take about six weeks to heal.

A strain is an injury in which muscle fibers have been pulled or damaged; pain is felt when the child moves the injured part on his own, but not when he relaxes and it is moved by someone else. Strains may take from days to weeks to heal.

Both sprains and strains cause pain and swelling. Bad ones make it hard or impossible to use the injured part. If a knee has been badly hurt, it should have a doctor's attention right away. Ankles can usually wait a few days, with home treatment, till some of the swelling goes down.

If, after a hard bump or fall, a child can't raise her arm on the hurt side and her shoulders look uneven, her collarbone (clavicle) may be broken. Children's collarbones are easily fractured; they are still forming and therefore partly cartilage. A child with a broken collarbone should see a doctor right away; collarbones usually heal in about a month, with only a protective brace as treatment.

Children's back and neck injuries are usually simple muscle strains from falls and accidents or adventurous acrobatics, but sometimes ligaments are damaged as well, or bones put out of place. The body has a tendency to guard its hurt parts from further pain by tightening the muscles around them so healing can take place without more aggravation. Sometimes, especially if the injury involves the neck, back, or pelvis, this guarding may lead to chronic muscular imbalances and spinal misalignments. A chiropractor, naturopath, or osteopath who uses low-force methods and is well experienced in treating children may be able to adjust the vertebrae (or extremities), restore muscular balance, and help with proper healing.

WHAT A PHYSICIAN MAY DO

A doctor will feel the joint with her fingertips and gently move it to find out where and how serious the injury is. If a fracture is suspected, X rays may be taken. Dislocated bones will be repositioned, and bandages, splints, or braces put on to keep the hurt part stable, and allow it to rest until it heals. If there is excessive swelling, the doctor may draw out some of the fluid with a needle.

Doctors will usually recommend aspirin for the pain. Since aspirin has been known to cause serious allergic reactions, it is better to use something safer (see below).

WHAT YOU CAN DO AT HOME

PRACTICAL MEASURES. First check for signs of a broken bone: Did the child hear a pop or crunch when the injury occurred? Is the pain and swelling extreme? Is it impossible for the child to move the limb or bear weight on it? If you think a bone might be broken, take the child to a doctor. (See FRACTURES.)

For a sprain or strain, apply ice wrapped in a damp towel to the injured place for at least twenty minutes, then take it off for ten, put it on again for twenty, and so on. Repeat this procedure several times during the day. Heat will increase the swelling, so do not let the child have a hot bath or apply any form of heat for at least forty-eight hours.

After the initial ice packs, use a comfrey poultice (leaves or roots softened in warm water and spread on a damp cloth, which is then wrapped around the injured part). Leave it on for several hours or overnight. Firm (but not too hard) pressure, as from an elastic bandage, can help control the swelling a bit. After the first forty-eight hours have passed, the hurt part may be soaked in warm water to which strong thyme or rosemary tea has been added.

Any action that hurts at all should be avoided. Sometimes wrappings, slings, or splints can keep the joint still enough to allow the child to do small things without reinjuring it.

Extra vitamins C, E, calcium, magnesium, and manganese may aid healing.

Occasionally, a reluctant-to-walk or wandering child will receive a firm pull on the arm, and the thumb-side bone of the forearm near the elbow can be displaced. Parents or babysitters may be abashed and embarrassed when this happens, but since the bone end is not yet fully formed not much force is needed to make it slip from its restraining ligament. *If the arm is not swollen or painful,* try the following procedure: With the child holding her arm with the palm turned downward, stabilize the elbow with one hand; with your other hand, move the forearm until it forms a right angle with the upper arm, then stretch the forearm gently away from the elbow, while turning the palm upward. If one or two gentle attempts at this do not realign the bone, seek help from a health care expert.

HOMEOPATHIC REMEDIES.

Arnica montana. Should be given as soon as possible to reduce the bruising and swelling. If the skin isn't broken, Arnica ointment can be rubbed into the hurt part several times a day.

Bryonia. Even slight motion increases the pain.

Ledum palustre. Sprained part is swollen but feels cold.

Rhus toxicodendron. Joint or muscle is stiff but feels better with gentle motion.

Ruta graveolens. Sprains and strains that are slow to get well, also for bone bruises.

TEETH AND GUMS
(see also MOUTH AND TONGUE)

The condition of a child's teeth is greatly affected by diet, hygiene, and heredity. A child who eats refined and processed foods and lots of sticky things (especially sugary ones) will be more inclined toward tooth decay, as will a baby whose mother was not well nourished during pregnancy. A child whose parents have a history of tooth problems is likely to have some trouble with his as well. Certain drugs (such as tetracycline) and other toxic substances, if taken by a pregnant woman, can cause the child's teeth to come in stained.

FLUORIDE

Fluoride is often prescribed as a supplement, and in many regions of the country it is added to the public water supply. Flourine (or its salt-form, fluoride) does not appear to be an essential nutrient, although it may—like other toxic minerals—be required by the body in extremely small amounts. There is evidence that fluoride incorporated into tooth structure helps the enamel resist decay; however, regular external exposure (as in toothpaste or fluoride rinses) seems to accomplish this without ingestion.

Fluoride, in similar concentrations to that in fluoridated public water, has been shown to inhibit the action of enzymes, cause chromosome-damage, birth defects, and miscarriages in studies with animals. Degeneration of the heart and arteries, and tissues of other vital organs including the kidneys, liver, pancreas and brain have been associated with excess fluoride.

Certain individuals appear to be more sensitive to fluoride than others. Toxicity figures of 2 to 5 grams (at which point tooth mottling or weakening are seen) are often cited by dentists and doctors—but cases of death and serious illness occurred in adults and children from doses much lower than these. A 250 microgram dose of fluoride has caused acute poisoning in babies; a dose of 500 micrograms has caused hemorrhage in the digestive system. Children have died from toxicity after dental fluoride-treatments. Toxic symptoms of fluoride may be mottled teeth, brittle or deformed bones and teeth, arthritis, calcification of soft tissues (including arteries), and problems in the kidneys, digestive system, heart, pancreas, liver, brain, and most of the vital organs of the body. Allergic reactions to fluoride may include rashes, weakness, nausea, vomiting, bleeding, and disability. Persons with certain kidney disorders can die from ingestion of tiny amounts of fluoride.

The body stores fluoride in its tissues, and people exposed to very low levels over time can experience toxic effects. Fluoride is a widespread industrial pollutant (the form used in public water-fluoridation programs seems often to have been obtained through purchase of industrial waste), and is now widely found in air and water, often causing serious toxic symptoms. Use of fluoridated water in commercial food processing, and the addition of fluoride to toothpastes and children's vitamin supplements contribute to the overall fluoride intake.

Research suggests that fluoride is more a toxic chemical than a nutrient, and that its intentional addition to much of the nation's drinking water may be increasing the risk of cancer, heart disease, and unhealthy genetic changes. Many researchers and citizens feel that the supplementation of fluoride should be a matter of choice and not imposed upon them—especially in light of the fact that many nutrients known to be more necessary to the body (and much less toxic) are regulated or restricted by the government.

TEETHING

A baby's teeth begin to form well before birth, but they don't start pushing out through the gums until about four months of age. Then at intervals until age two or later, teething episodes occur. Some babies feel miserable during teething; some don't seem to mind it too much, although it always hurts. The baby may be cranky, drool excessively, have a runny nose, refuse to eat or nurse, and want to bite down hard on any available object. During teething, a substance present in the baby's saliva can cause a rash on his chin and neck. Bowel movements may be smellier and more likely to cause redness.

Teething gels or lotions containing anesthetics should be avoided; these drugs can cause a serious allergic reaction. Aspirin, acetaminophen, and other drugs should not be used.

Fever or real illness (except diarrhea, or occasional spitting up due to excess saliva) can't be caused by teething. However, since it is a time of stress, the child's resistance to disease may be lowered. Any real illness should be considered and treated in its own right, and not written off as "just teething."

WHAT YOU CAN DO AT HOME

PRACTICAL MEASURES. Give a teething child cold, hard things to chew on—for example, a hard rubber toy kept in the freezer, an ice cube wrapped in a cloth, a big solid carrot stick. Choose these according to the child's age, so there is no danger of choking on dislodged bits of food or broken bits of toys.

To soothe the pain, one part clove oil may be mixed with four parts olive oil and rubbed on the gums. Test it on your own gums first; if it burns, add more olive oil.

HERB TEAS. Chamomile, lemon balm.

HOMEOPATHIC REMEDIES.
> *Belladonna.* Baby is flushed and restless, may seem to have little fits or be easily startled from sleep.
> *Calcarea carbonica.* Teeth take a long time to come in; child may be chubby, easily tired.
> *Calcarea phosphorica.* Teeth come in late; child may be thin, and like bacon and junk foods.
> *Chamomilla.* Baby is very irritable, screams and throws things;

pain almost unbearable; better from cold, pressure, and being carried.

Coffea. Baby seems very excitable and can't sleep.

Ignatia. Baby seems sad, sighs, has flushes of heat; limbs may jerk during sleep.

Sulphur. Whitish, burning diarrhea or peeling rash accompanies teething.

TOOTH DECAY

A coating of sugars and starches from food left on or between the teeth can support bacteria; these multiply and produce an acid that destroys enamel. After the enamel is demineralized, causing cavities, the inner part of the tooth may also become infected. Children should visit a dentist if their teeth hurt or appear discolored or any cavities are visible. Checkups with a dentist once a year or more are often recommended, although children who take good care of their teeth and are well nourished may not need to go this often.

As soon as a child has teeth, daily brushing should begin. Parents have to do this at first, of course. After the child shows an interest in doing it herself (about age two or three), parents should follow up to clean the missed places. Show her how to find all the surfaces—front, back, top, bottom, while opening wide or clenching the teeth to reach the different spots. Children are usually not thorough brushers until the age of four or older, but it is good to get them into the habit of brushing their teeth themselves. Once a day is usually enough, although extra brushing or rinsing the mouth after sweets or sticky foods should be encouraged.

Flossing (once there are enough teeth close together to floss between) can get rid of tiny bits of trapped food that might start cavities. Waxed and flavored flosses can be used to make this process more appealing.

Many toothpastes have too strong a flavor for babies, but milder brands can be found in natural food stores. Some natural health advocates recommend brushing with sea salt, baking soda, or charcoal powder; successful use of these depends upon the brusher's age and tastes. To remove yellow stains, a fresh strawberry may be put on the brush and used as toothpaste, then left on for fifteen minutes. Teeth and gums can be invigorated by rubbing them up and down with lemon or lime peel.

To strengthen the child against tooth decay, make sure he gets good-quality protein every day and eats fresh fruits and vegetables and whole-grain foods rather than refined foods and sweets. Foods especially healthful for teeth and gums include sesame seeds, barley, fresh parsley, kelp, and alfalfa sprouts. A balanced vitamin and mineral supplement taken every day is helpful. Avoiding sugar and sticky foods is a good idea. Until a child is three or four, parents may find it possible to keep the existence of candy a secret; after that it is very difficult. Children (and parents) should eat desserts or candy only as very special treats. Keep fresh fruits, berries, and canned unsweetened pineapple on hand to satisfy a sweet tooth. Honey and dried fruits are nutritionally preferable to refined sugar and candy, but they can stick to teeth and cause decay.

Eating hard, raw fruits and vegetables at the end of a meal can clean the teeth. Cheese is said to contain an enzyme that fights tooth decay, which may explain why in some parts of the world it is customary to serve cheese for dessert.

Vitamins C, A, D, B-complex (especially B_6, folic acid, niacinamide, and pantothenic acid), calcium, and magnesium can help a child's teeth grow strong and resist decay.

TOOTHACHES

If a child has a toothache, and you can see a hole or brown spot in his tooth, you can be fairly sure that this is the cause of the pain. Sometimes a cavity in a tooth will cause the gums to be sore and red or the whole jaw to swell. If there is an abscess, it may be accompanied by fever. Toothaches do not always come from teeth; sometimes the pain from a nasal, sinus, or throat infection extends to the teeth. Teeth can also ache from muscle tension, neck misalignment, or gum irritation or inflammation. If you suspect that your child has a cavity, or tooth pain persists in a particular area, take him to the dentist as soon as you can get an appointment.

WHAT A DENTIST MAY DO

The dentist will examine the teeth and probe with instruments to discover the location and extent of cavities and decay. Many dentists like to take X rays in order to have a quick, convenient view of the state of the teeth. Since repeated exposure is harmful, you should ask the dentist either to work without X rays, or to limit them to those that are absolutely essential. Make sure a lead apron and all possible shielding is used to protect your child. If a child has an upcoming appointment with the dentist, especially if X rays are expected, give him extra vitamin C, E, and kelp (all of which help protect against radiation) for several days. Some dentists use natural, less toxic methods of treatment, including homeopathic remedies.

WHAT YOU CAN DO AT HOME

Biting down with the sore tooth on a whole clove or applying a swab dipped in oil of cloves can numb the pain, although some children dislike how "hot" it feels. A few grains of cayenne pepper may be applied to the aching or inflamed tooth and gum. Fresh aloe vera juice may be rubbed on the gums and put in the cavity. Dental floss may be used to remove jammed food on both sides and around the affected tooth. Vitamins C and E can help make gums less sensitive and inflamed.

HOMEOPATHIC REMEDIES.

Aconitum napellus. Face feels hot; child is frantic with pain or fear; sudden onset, often after exposure to cold and wind.

Antimonium crudum. Child's teeth are rotten and discolored; pain often comes from several teeth at once.

Belladonna. Cutting pain in the roots of the teeth on biting down; heat and throbbing; child is very restless; hard pressure on the cheek may ease the pain.

Chamomilla. Pain is extreme and makes the child irritable and angry; worse during the night; it may be unclear which tooth is causing the ache.

Mercurius vivus. Ache comes from decayed teeth; swollen gums; stinging or wrenching pains that send stitches into the head; worse from damp, cold air; rubbing the cheek may help.

Pulsatilla. Child is weepy and wants constantly to be comforted; toothache may be accompanied by earache.

Homeopathic remedies may also help a nervous child before a dental appointment, and to curb pain afterward:

Arnica montana. Before a dental appointment, to reduce bruising of the gums, and after dental work if the tooth is very sore.

Chamomilla. If child is extra-sensitive to pain.
Gelsemium. If child feels shaky, nervous, fearful, or has
diarrhea.

ACUPRESSURE AND MASSAGE.
- For pain in upper teeth: tender spots in face muscles just in front of
  the jaw joint.
- For pain in lower teeth: tender spots at the angle of the jaw.
  LI 4: The point at the end of the crease between the thumb and
  index finger. Hold these points, on both hands at the same time,
  for several minutes.
  LV 3: A tender point midway between the first and second metatarsal bones.
  ST 45: The point on the second toe at the edge of the nail bed nearest the foot and the middle toe.

TOOTH-GRINDING

A child who grinds her teeth is likely to be under some sort of
nervous stress. This may have an emotional cause such as anxiety
about family or school, or the stress may be a physical one such as
allergy or nutritional deficiency. If the child habitually fidgets,
picks her nose, scratches her bottom, and sucks her thumb past
the age of three, the tooth-grinding may be due to worms (see
WORMS).

WHAT YOU CAN DO AT HOME

PRACTICAL MEASURES. Try to find out, without making the child
feel put on the spot, what her feelings are and what might be distressing her. Bedtime is a good occasion for a relaxed talk and
backrub; during the day, having a tea party or taking a walk together may be a good time for sharing confidences.

Remove refined and processed foods (especially sugar) from
the child's diet. Give her a high-protein snack half an hour before bedtime to help her blood-sugar level stay steady during the
night.

Supplements of calcium and magnesium, vitamin C, and balanced B-complex with extra pantothenic acid can help calm the
nerves and help deal with stress.

Spinal or cranial manipulations, given by specially trained dentists, orthodontists, chiropractors, naturopaths, osteopaths, and craniosacral therapists will help relieve nervous stress that leads to tooth-grinding.

THROAT INFLAMMATIONS

Sore throats are usually associated with cold viruses and strep or staph infections. There is often red swelling of the throat tissues and tonsils. The child may feel a lump, or pain extending into the ears, when swallowing. White patches on the tonsils, bad breath, and swollen lymph nodes in the neck may be symptoms of strep throat or mononucleosis.

If a child feels ill and feverish with a very sore throat but no runny nose, cough or other symptoms, strep throat is a possibility. Although strep throat usually makes a child more ill than a viral sore throat, most cases clear up with rest in several days; strep throat can lead to scarlet fever or kidney infection, but this is very rare. If the throat is terribly sore, or there is drooling and extreme difficulty in opening the mouth or swallowing, a doctor should check for strep involvement or abscess.

Sometimes the throat feels dry or scratchy from mild infection, allergy, too-dry air (as from electric heat), excessive use of the voice (shouting, crying, screaming, raucous singing), or breathing with the mouth open.

Laryngitis is inflammation of the larynx (voice box) causing loss of the voice or a hoarse change in the voice. It can be very mild and have no other symptoms, or it can be accompanied by sore throat, fever, and difficulty swallowing. Laryngitis may be associated with such maladies as bronchitis, flu, tonsilitis, sinusitis, whooping cough, and measles. Other causes of laryngitis are exposure to cigarette smoke, inhaling polluted air or noxious fumes, and overuse of the voice. If a child younger than three months old is hoarse or loses his voice for any length of time, he should be checked by a doctor, in case this is caused by a defect in the throat or cardiorespiratory system or a thyroid problem.

If any throat condition lasts for more than a week or there is real difficulty with breathing or swallowing, take the child to a doctor.

WHAT A PHYSICIAN MAY DO

The doctor will look into the throat using a light and tongue depressor to examine the tonsils and check for abscesses. A throat swab and culture to test for strep involvement may be taken. (Note: Streptococcus bacteria are present in the throats of some people whether they are sick or not. A positive strep test does not always mean a strep infection.) Some doctors suspecting infection give antibiotics, even without a positive strep culture. Unless an infection is very severe and the child is miserable, these are better avoided and natural remedies used instead.

Sore throats caused by mononucleosis may last many weeks. Doctors can diagnose mononucleosis by means of a blood test, but usually provide no further treatment than recommending good nutrition and rest.

WHAT YOU CAN DO AT HOME

PRACTICAL MEASURES. Honey and lemon juice mixed together can make a soothing syrup. Sucking on slippery-elm lozenges, zinc lozenges, vitamin C tablets, or herbal cough drops may ease the soreness. (Avoid eucalyptus, camphor, or strong aromatic substances if homeopathic remedies are being used.)

Gargling can relieve hoarseness, pain, and swelling. Use cider vinegar in hot water (two tablespoons to half a cup), hot salt water (a teaspoon of salt dissolved in one-half cup water), or lemon juice.

Include lots of clear liquids and fruit in the diet. Garlic, onions, and horseradish can help fight infection. Extra vitamins A, C, and zinc will also help.

HERB TEAS. Echinacea, comfrey, licorice root, slippery elm, peppermint, red clover, dillweed, coltsfoot.

HOMEOPATHIC REMEDIES. (See also TONSILS AND ADENOIDS.)
Aconitum napellus. Sore throat that comes on suddenly with pricking, burning pain, fever, great anxiety.
Belladonna. Very red throat, worse on the right; child is hot, flushed, feverish, with throbbing headache.
Hepar sulphuris calcareum. Hoarseness; pain like a splinter on

swallowing, extends to ears; child is easily irritated, has chills, sweats; worse from cold air and drafts

Ignatia. Child feels a lump or sore spot in the throat, which may be relieved by swallowing; swollen or ulcerated tonsils; after grief or emotional upsets.

Lycopodium. Throat sore on the right side (or may begin on the right and move to the left); relief from warm drinks; worse from 4:00 to 8:00 P.M.; child may have gas and feel tired, not really ill.

Mercurius vivus. Throat swollen, tonsils may have yellow or white patches on them; coated tongue; fever, chills, difficulty swallowing; worse at night; child may drool in sleep.

Phosphorus. Larynx feels raw and painful, talking causes violent tickling; worse in the evening; child is thirsty for cold drinks, likes to be rubbed.

Rhus toxicodendron. Painful throat, better from warmth and motion; child feels worse in the morning.

Spongia tosta. Hoarseness, larynx tender to touch; dry, burning feeling in throat; child is worse before midnight; better lying down with head low.

Sulphur. Throat feels dry and burning, is better from warm drinks; sore throat keeps coming back.

Cistus canadensis. May be helpful if the sore throat is associated with mononucleosis.

ACUPRESSURE AND MASSAGE.

LI 4: The point at the end of the crease between the thumb and index finger.

LI 11: A tender point at the thumb-side end of the elbow-crease when the arm is bent.

LU 7: The tender point on the undersurface of the thumb-side forearm bone, two of the child's thumb-widths above the palm-side wrist-crease.

CV 22: A point in the notch at the base of the throat, just above the breastbone.

GV 14: The point at the tip of the big bump in the spine where the neck and upper back meet.

- A point at the middle of the wrist, just behind the back of the hand.
- Massage the neck muscles, front and back, concentrating on tender points.
- Rub the ring-finger side of the large knuckle where the middle finger joins the back of the hand.

TONSILS AND ADENOIDS

The tonsils are located on either side of the throat, just above the root of the tongue. The adenoids are found near the back of the nasal passages, at the openings of the eustachian tubes (which lead into the ears). They are all made of lymphatic tissue, which serves as defense against infection; while doing this work, the tonsils and adenoids may become enlarged—or infected themselves—in an attempt to save more important parts of the body from disease.

Most children between the ages of three and twelve have fairly large tonsils because they are constantly being exposed to viruses and infections to which their body has not yet formed immunity. Moderate tonsil enlargement, without pain or other symptoms, is not a cause for great concern; it means the immune system is doing its best to keep the child healthy. However, if the size of tonsils or adenoids interferes with breathing or swallowing, something has to be done to reduce their work load.

Allergy, particularly to dairy products, is a frequent offender. (See ALLERGIES.)

TONSILLITIS

Every time there is a throat infection, the tonsils (unless they've been removed) are involved to some degree. But during acute tonsillitis they may become severely inflamed, painful, and covered with yellow or white material. Acute tonsillitis is usually accompanied by high fever, chills, headache, stiff neck, sore tongue, and a feeling of fatigue and misery. The body usually overcomes the infection within a few days; if the symptoms last for a week or more, strep bacteria may be involved. (See THROAT INFLAMMATIONS.)

ADENOIDITIS

The adenoids, because of their location near the openings of the eustachian tubes and the internal junction of the nose and throat, have a tendency when swollen to cause blockage of the middle ear, loss of the senses of smell and taste, bad breath, and mental dullness caused by a decreased supply of oxygen to the brain. Children who are mouth-breathers, with a dull facial expression, nasal speech, diminished hearing, and bad breath, are likely to have enlarged adenoids.

WHAT A PHYSICIAN MAY DO

After examining the throat, and possibly doing a throat culture to check for strep, a doctor will probably prescribe antibiotics.

Removal of the tonsils and/or adenoids may be recommended if they are continually infected, or enlarged to the point that they actually obstruct breathing and contribute to enlargment of the heart because of the extra effort required to provide oxygen to all parts of the body. At one time, children's tonsils were taken out almost as a matter of course. Doctors, misunderstanding the tonsils' function, thought that the tonsils were a weak point, or even a source of disease, because of their tendency to become swollen. Because of this, many people were deprived of a valuable component of the immune system. Since tonsils and adenoids are a first line of defense against infection, their removal diverts the stress of disease toward more vital parts of the body. People whose tonsils have been taken out often go on to develop asthma or serious allergies and are more inclined to chronic ill health. Because of this danger, it is important that the child's whole body be strengthened against the infection and stress that chronic tonsillitis and adenoiditis indicate.

WHAT YOU CAN DO AT HOME

PRACTICAL MEASURES AND NUTRITION. The diet should be clean and light—fresh fruit and vegetable juices, or broths. Dairy products should be stopped, as should meats and refined or fatty foods. A child should receive a balanced daily vitamin-mineral supplement along with extra vitamins C, A, E, B-complex including pantothenic acid, and zinc.

Gargling with hot salt water, echinacea tea, a brew of goldenseal, or lemon juice, as well as sucking on vitamin C or acidophilus tablets throughout the day, can be soothing and help to fight the infection.

HERB TEAS. Echinacea, licorice root, slippery elm.

HOMEOPATHIC REMEDIES. (See also THROAT INFLAMMATIONS, INFECTIONS, and FEVER.)

>*Apis mellifica.* Tonsils are very swollen and rosy pink with white spots; pain has a stinging quality; better from cold drinks and food; child is not thirsty.

Belladonna. Bright red throat, worse on the right; throat feels dry and tight; swallowing liquids hurts; child may have high fever, red face; light hurts the eyes.

Calcarea phosphorica. Chronically enlarged tonsils that look pale and flabby; child may always seem dissatisfied, and crave bacon, sausages, junk food.

Ferrum phosphoricum. Red swelling of tonsils; tonsillitis recurs frequently; child has rosy cheeks and slight fever; worse at night and early morning.

Hepar sulphuris calcareum. Tonsils have white or yellow spots; sticking pains going into the ear are left on swallowing; child feels irritable, chilly, worse from drafts.

Mercurius vivus. Throat very sore, raw, infected, bluish-red swelling; lymph nodes in neck are swollen and tender; child may drool, sweat profusely, have bad breath.

Phytolacca. Tonsils look swollen and dark, especially on right; throat feels hot and narrow, worse from hot liquids; pain at the root of the tongue, shooting into the ears on swallowing; child feels worse in damp weather and from moving around.

Silicea. Chronic tonsillitis, abscesses in throat, stabbing pains like pinpricks; hard, swollen lymph nodes in neck; child may be delicate, easily tired.

For acupressure and massage, see THROAT INFLAMMATIONS.

URINARY TRACT CONDITIONS

Most problems involving the urinary tracts of small children are associated with bladder control. After the age of eighteen months, most children are aware that they are urinating and can begin to develop conscious control. This is usually achieved by the age of two and a half or three (see BEDWETTING).

If a newborn baby seems to need to push to get urine out, and does not have a good, strong stream, it may be that the passage from the bladder to the outside of the body is too small or obstructed. A doctor should check this, and enlarge the opening if necessary.

If an older child passes only a small amount of dark urine, or if the urine burns, it may be that she is not getting enough to drink. This happens frequently during hot weather, or illness with fever. Disorders of the bladder or kidneys may also cause this trouble.

Scanty, dark yellow urine, vomiting, diarrhea, excessive sweating, fever, loss of skin elasticity, sunken eyes, and headache are signs of dehydration. Very frequent urination along with excessive thirst, shortness of breath, nausea, vomiting, or coma may be signs of diabetes. (See DEHYDRATION and DIABETES.)

Sometimes there is a sore spot at the urinary opening (in girls, between the labia, just in front of the vagina; in boys, at the tip of the penis) that makes the urine sting as it comes out, or causes slight bleeding. This occurs more commonly in girls, and usually comes from improper wiping after bowel movements (proper wiping should be done front to back, not back to front); other causes may be sexual intercourse (in girls); foreign objects; dehydration; allergy; reactions to soaps, laundry detergents, bubble baths, toxic substances, or medicines; or emotional stress. Tight clothing or synthetic fabrics that do not allow the skin to breathe may make infection more likely.

Occasionally, a child will have a kidney or bladder infection. If serious, these are often accompanied by other symptoms such as fever, discharge, nausea, vomiting, back pain, and abdominal pain.

BLADDER INFECTION (Cystitis)
The main symptom of bladder infection is frequent, urgent, sometimes painful urination; occasionally there is a feeling of general illness, and a small amount of blood or pus may be seen in the urine. Bladder infections can usually be controlled by home measures (see below), but if the discomfort is severe, a doctor can give medication to help relieve it.

KIDNEY INFECTION (Nephritis)
During a kidney infection, a child may experience some of these symptoms: fever, shaking chills; pain when urinating, strong or putrid-smelling, dark, smoky, or pink-colored urine that may contain pus; headache; unexplained pains in the abdomen, groin, or

back; nausea; swelling of the face and ankles. Sometimes kidney involvement follows a condition involving strep or staph bacteria, such as strep throat or impetigo. It is wise to consult a physician right away if there is any suspicion that the kidneys are involved; although these infections are often mild and short-lasting, they can be very serious.

WHAT A PHYSICIAN MAY DO

A urine sample will most likely be taken, and the doctor will examine the abdomen, back, urinary openings, and genital areas. Sometimes an X ray, or even hospital observation, may be recommended if the kidney involvement seems severe. Doctors usually prescribe ampicillin or sulfa drugs, which can have serious side effects. As in all diseases, drugs should be used only if the disease is very severe and cannot be controlled by natural therapies.

WHAT YOU CAN DO AT HOME

PRACTICAL MEASURES AND NUTRITION. Make a poultice of fresh crushed comfrey leaves wrapped in a light cotton cloth, and apply it to the painful areas (usually abdomen or back).

Have the child drink plenty of fluids (avoiding citrus juices). Cranberry juice is beneficial because it contains a substance that has an antibacterial effect in the body. Use a brand that is not sugar-sweetened. Eating lots of watermelon, including the seeds, helps cleanse the urinary tract. Other foods thought to benefit the kidneys are goat's milk, papayas, bananas, cucumbers, eggplant, asparagus, watercress, onions, garlic, horseradish, and flaxseed.

Balanced B-complex vitamins, including adequate choline, B_{12}, and folic acid, as well as vitamins C, A, and E are especially helpful. (Dr. Lendon Smith says that taking 100–500 mg. of vitamin C per hour will keep the urine acidic and inhospitable to bacteria.)

HERB TEAS. Buchu, parsley, cornsilk, red raspberry leaf, rose hips, dandelion, comfrey, juniper berry, oatstraw, fennel.

HOMEOPATHIC REMEDIES.
> *Aconitum napellus.* Urine is suddenly retained, after anxiety, fear, or being chilled.

Apis mellifica. Stinging, scanty urination, worse from heat; abdominal tenderness, fever.

Cantharis. Burning pain, strong urge but only a few drops pass; backache.

Mercurius vivus. Strong urge, burning pain, small amounts of dark urine; worse at night; child may sweat, drool in sleep, have swollen glands, bad breath.

Nux vomica. Strong, frequent, painful urge to urinate but little comes out; child may be pushy, irritable, chilly.

Pulsatilla. Strong urging, worse from lying on back; child is sweet, weepy, worse in warm room and from heat.

Staphysagria. Pressure in bladder, feeling of a drop of urine always in the channel; child may be very sensitive, easily hurt and embarrassed.

Thuja. Frequent painful urination; sudden urge; child has to get up a lot in the night; urine has very strong odor.

ACUPRESSURE AND MASSAGE.

KI 3: The tender point just behind the upper rear aspect of the inner anklebone.

LV 3: A tender point midway between the first and second metatarsal bones.

BL 60: A tender point in the hollow behind the outer anklebone, in front of the Achilles tendon.

LI 4: The point at the end of the crease between the thumb and index finger.

WEIGHT PROBLEMS

There is no ideal weight for children of a certain size or age. The shape of the child's body has much to do with heredity and the growing process, not only with physical fitness and eating habits. Certain children go through chubby phases without having a real weight problem; a pudgy period may be followed by a spurt in height that evens everything out. Many children, especially while growing rapidly, may appear to be extremely skinny even while eating constantly. Some children seem to eat practically nothing for long periods of time, yet their weight remains about the same. Some people are naturally stockier than others, some have bigger waists or legs or bottoms. It is likely that a child is overweight if significant rolls of fat are seen anywhere, or if exercise seems difficult because the child has to haul extra pounds around. If a thin child seems weak and listless, very nervous, or looks extremely emaciated, the condition needs attention. To decide whether a child's weight is normal, her appearance and energy level should be considered, not the number on the scales. Observe her overall strength, health, and brightness. If she is alert, happy, interested in things, physically energetic, and has good resistance to illness, there is usually little need to worry. It is important, however, that her diet is healthy and includes the necessary nutrients for growth.

There are things parents can do to help prevent weight problems from developing in their children. Children should not be forced to eat if they're not hungry, to always clean their plates, or to eat foods they really don't like. Children should be encouraged to respond to their body's natural hunger cues; as long as junk-food isn't easily accessible, they will naturally regulate their eating unless they are lacking certain nutrients. Don't let eating become an emotional issue; have healthy foods available, but let children make their own decisions about when and what to eat. Encourage them to exercise (by walking, hiking, bicycling and playing outdoor games with them) and set a good example by eating prudently yourself. Do not let your children be distressed or pressured by society's neurotic emphasis of having a "perfect" body.

WHAT A PHYSICIAN MAY DO

A doctor may perform a full physical examination as well as checking for allergies, nutritional deficiencies, or absorption problems. Tests may be done to check thyroid function and hormonal status. Dietary and psychological factors will be considered. A doctor may prescribe a particular diet, encourage regular exercise, give supplements or medications (such as thyroid hormone) or refer the child for psychiatric help or counseling.

OVERWEIGHT

Obesity can be a damaging condition, physically and psychologically. A fat child may find his life crippled by self-consciousness, and may miss out on necessary play and friendship because of his clumsiness. His heart may be under physical strain as well, and the development of coordination may be slowed.

Forcefully cutting down the amount a child eats is *not* the best solution to a weight problem. It is hard to deny a hungry child food. Not only is it pleasant and comforting to eat, but feeling hungry is usually a signal that the child's growing body needs something. *What* the child's body needs is the question that should most concern you. If she is in the habit of eating nonnutritious foods (fried or processed foods, desserts, candy), she may turn to such things every time her body is asking for nourishment. If parents willingly supply nonnutritious, addictive foods, they may have fat, malnourished children on their hands.

Do not allow a child (or anyone) to use weight-loss pills. These can be damaging, and extremely so to a body that is still growing. Some of these pills are diuretics, which achieve weight reduction not by encouraging the burning of fat but by removing water from the body. The "lost" weight is replaced as soon as the water is replenished, and the diuretic action on the body tissues (and consequent dehydration) can cause many problems. Other diet pills may contain amphetamines to speed up metabolism and burn off fat. These are extremely dangerous drugs. Parents who allow their child to take them are either ignorant or irresponsible.

WHAT YOU CAN DO AT HOME

PRACTICAL MEASURES AND NUTRITION. A good solution is to find healthful foods that the child likes. The easiest way to do this is to start him out, as a baby, on rice cakes, raw carrots, or slices of fruit for treats—closely guarding the secret that sugar and junk foods exist. (This usually only works for a year or two, depending on how well you train the siblings and grandparents.) Many children do prefer fruit to candy, and lightly sweetened granola to cloying puddings—but many adults (who may personally think of junk foods as treats) do not always understand this. Most desserts, especially pies and cookies, can be baked at home, using half the usual sweetening (in the form of fruit syrups or honey instead of sugar), and whole-grain or unrefined flours; these simple changes can transform a fattening food into a nutritious (and often more palatable) one.

Children who have food allergies and are on restricted diets to help overcome health problems such as stomachaches or asthma are often very cooperative about sticking to their regimen. This may be partly because the children want to avoid the episodes of feeling ill that follow eating the forbidden foods . . . but it might also be because the *parents* are more diligent about providing good foods when they know that the child is allergic to something.

Practically everyone is "allergic" to foods that are loaded with sugar and fat—feeling run-down and slumpy after eating them. Such foods eaten in excess are known to contribute to heart and artery disease and diabetes. So, if you want to tell people that your child has an "intolerance" to refined and processed foods, you will not be stretching the truth.

A nourishing diet and an adequate supply of vitamins and minerals may keep a child from overeating or craving unhealthy foods. Foods that children often like that will help with weight loss include: grapefruit, apples, cherries, pineapple, carrots, celery, cabbage, lettuce, cucumbers, radishes, and alfalfa sprouts. Give whole grains rather than refined flour, and lean, low-fat protein foods such as yogurt, fresh fish, and skinless chicken or turkey. A child's diet should not be completely fat-free, because certain fatty acids are essential nutrients for growth and health. In fact, a small amount of oil in the diet—a tablespoon a day or so—is necessary for the efficient metabolism of fat. Cold-pressed sunflower and sesame oils are two of the most healthful.

Nutritional supplements, taken daily, may help the body convert its fat to energy. Balanced B-complex with choline and inositol, lecithin, calcium, magnesium, vitamins E and C, and kelp are especially helpful.

HERB TEAS. Kelp, chickweed, nettle, Irish moss.

UNDERWEIGHT

If the child looks emaciated, or is very thin, with a protuberant abdomen, and does not seem very healthy, the reasons must be considered: Does she seem to eat plenty and still fail to gain weight? It may be that her body is not properly absorbing food. When this is the case, bowel movements are usually abnormal—they may be too bulky, too loose, look greasy, or smell foul. Inadequate absorption of food may be caused by food allergy. (Celiac disease, an absorption disorder, is related to an allergy to gluten, a substance found in wheat, oats, and rye.)

Some factors that may contribute to insufficient weight gain are: a lack of necessary digestive enzymes, improper chewing, incompatible food combinations, vitamin and mineral deficiencies, intestinal parasites (see WORMS), and emotional stress. Thyroid disorders or anorexia and bulimia (see below) may also contribute to unhealthy loss of weight.

WHAT YOU CAN DO AT HOME

PRACTICAL MEASURES AND NUTRITION. Do not give the child large quantities of fattening foods in hopes of raising the reading on the scales. What matters is health, not poundage. In fact, it is probably best to stay away from scales completely. Do not limit the child's eating to mealtimes—let him have frequent snacks, and keep nutritious foods he likes on hand at all times. Fruit, cheese, yogurt, celery and peanut butter, whole-grain crackers, and granola are good choices. Don't insist that he eat things he doesn't like. This may be difficult, as some children claim to like nothing but junk food. Luckily, natural food stores are beginning to have some very palatable snacks—cookies sweetened with rice syrup or fruit juice; soy milk shakes; nonsugar ice cream and frozen yogurt; whole-grain chips, pretzels, and corn curls—most of which are more nutritious than their empty-calorie counter-parts.

Provide plenty of fresh fruit and vegetables, whole grains (especially barley), and good-quality protein. Foods that contain essential fatty acids, such as wheat germ, soy products, and sunflower and sesame seeds, may stimulate the appetite.

Be sure the child takes good-quality vitamin and mineral supplements every day, with extra B-complex and zinc.

An undernourished child should be encouraged to eat but not made to feel nervous about it. Some children may become stubborn about eating, because they've been made to feel self-conscious about being skinny, and exert their will by having a contrary reaction. Some children (especially teenagers) get it into their minds that they are fat, even if they are not, and starve themselves.

Anorexia nervosa is a serious condition, in which a child or teenager (most often female) becomes preoccupied with food but obsessively refuses to eat. This can bring about severe weight loss, and consequent loss of menstrual periods and other endocrine problems. *Bulimia* is a tendency for a child to overeat in binges, then make herself vomit, use laxatives, weight-loss pills, or diuretics to try to purge and keep from gaining weight. This can be very dangerous, as mineral balance in the body can be seriously altered by these practices.

These eating disorders often seem to be related to deep fear and unhappiness, sometimes to a fear of maturing sexually. If a child appears to be nervous or unhappy about something in her life, try to get her to talk about it with a parent or other trusted adult. Children with such problems often need professional counseling. Choose a counselor carefully: be certain that the child is comfortable talking with this person, and that drugs (or other techniques that suppress or increase the stress without truly relieving the problem) are not used.

WHOOPING COUGH (Pertussis)

Whooping cough is an exhausting disease, particularly dangerous for children under two years old. It is transmitted via airborne droplets, and very contagious. Attacks of whooping cough in some children, especially older ones, may be mild; some experts think that many unrecognized or unreported cases occur. A number of children who contract whooping cough have received all recommended doses of the vaccine against it (the pertussis element of the DPT shot; see the chapter on Immunizations). Symptoms of whooping cough in "immunized" children may not fit the typical description and therefore may not be recognized.

The first symptoms occur one to two weeks after exposure, beginning with a fairly mild cough that is usually, but not always accompanied by typical cold symptoms. Gradually the cough gets worse until the child experiences bouts of coughing—repeated long strings of coughs, with a "whooping" gasp for air between jags. Thick phlegm may cause choking, and the child can swallow large amounts of it, which are later vomited. Paroxysms may be started by laughing, breathing cold air, or exertion. (Small babies, who are less accustomed to breathing efficiently, may choke rather than make the "whooping" sound; they often vomit and may appear blue-gray from lack of oxygen. A baby with such symptoms needs immediate medical attention.)

The most severe phase of the illness usually lasts about two weeks, with another two weeks or so of convalescence. Any child with whooping cough should be kept away from other children, especially babies and toddlers, for at least four weeks. It is important in any severe case of whooping cough, and especially with a child under two, to get a doctor's help as soon as the disease is suspected.

WHAT A PHYSICIAN MAY DO
Whooping cough can be diagnosed by bacterial culture (taken from a nose-and-throat swab) or a blood test. In the early stages, a doctor may prescribe antibiotics or pertussis immune globulin (for children under the age of two) in hopes of preventing complications. If the child is very small, is having tremendous difficulty breathing, or is greatly exhausted, the doctor may advise keeping him in the hospital, where breathing support can be given and lost fluids and nutrients replaced.

WHAT YOU CAN DO AT HOME
Constant watching, nursing, and reassurance are indispensible; the child should never be left alone, as the coughing and breathing difficulty can be frightening, and inhaling vomited material is potentially fatal if no one is there to help.

Tiny sips of fluids or small amounts of light food should be given soon after each coughing paroxysm subsides, so the child does not become weak or dehydrated.

Poultices of crushed garlic cloves wrapped in a cotton cloth and applied to the soles of the feet are helpful in some cases.

HERB TEAS. Coltsfoot, horehound, thyme, violet flower, black currant leaves, ginger, sage, wild cherry bark.

HOMEOPATHIC REMEDIES. (See also COUGH.) If you think that a child has been exposed to whooping cough, giving the remedy *Corallium* in a 30C potency may prevent an attack or make it milder.

Antimonium tartaricum. Wet, rattling sounds from mucus in the chest; whitecoated tongue; diarrhea; vomiting after midnight; worse from warm drinks; child needs to sit up to keep from suffocating.

Arnica montana. Child may dread the coming cough and cry before it begins; violent spasms of coughing, made worse by anger.

Belladonna. Tickling in the thoat; deep, hollow, dry cough may cause bloodshot eyes or nosebleed; pain in head and stomach; red face; child may clutch her throat, be frightened.

Carbo vegetabilis. Burning pain in the chest after coughing; gagging and vomiting up lumps of phlegm; child sweats but feels cold, wants moving air, windows open.

Cuprum metallicum. Violent coughing fits with convulsions, prostration; cramping in toes and fingers.

Drosera. Very deep, hoarse coughing jags, worse after midnight; chest feels oppressed; breathing is very difficult and painful. This remedy is said to work best when given only once, in the 30C potency.

Ipecacuanha. Violent spells of coughing, with little chance for breathing between them; much nausea and vomiting; child's body stiffens and complexion may turn bluish.

Veratrum album. Hollow cough that comes on after cold drinks or exposure to cold air; child feels cold, looks blue, with cold sweat, weak pulse, abdominal pain.

ACUPRESSURE AND MASSAGE.

LU 1: A tender point in the indentation below the shoulder end of the collarbone.

LI 4: The point at the end of the crease between the thumb and index finger.

ST 36: A tender point next to the outer side of the big bump at the top of the shin.

SP 6: A tender point three of the child's finger-breadths above the inner anklebone.

CV 22: A point in the notch at the base of the throat, just above the breastbone.

· A point in the pad of the hand below the crack between index and middle fingers.

· Massage the muscles of the upper back, along the spine.

· Massage the muscles along the tops of the shoulders.

WORMS

Different types of intestinal parasites may enter children's bodies; these vary according to sanitation, environment, and climate. Poor hygiene, malnutrition, unsanitary eating habits, and contact with manure or animals are contributing causes. The most ubiquitous (and innocuous) of such parasites is the pinworm, which can be caught by almost anyone. Other types of worms, such as roundworm, hookworm, and tapeworm, can cause more serious health problems.

PINWORMS (Seatworms, Enterobiasis)

These worms are quite common visitors to children, even those with fairly clean habits. A child with pinworms may scratch his itchy bottom and, carrying the minuscule eggs under his fingernails, can then transfer them to food or objects from which they are passed on to other people. Bad breath, dark circles around the eyes, pallor around the mouth, coughing, nose-picking, toothgrinding, and waking in the night with pain or itching around the anus or rectum suggest their presence. Complications from pinworms include irritated or infected areas of skin from scratching and vaginal irritation from migrating worms.

Pinworms can be detected on a sleeping child by looking at the area around the anus with a flashlight several hours after bedtime, when the female worms crawl out to lay their eggs. Or a bit of cellophane tape can be touched over the hole, and worms or eggs picked up. The worms look like short white threads, about a quarter-inch long. If the child (and parents) exercise scrupulous cleanliness, pinworms can go away without medication within several weeks. Natural treatments often safely speed this process.

ROUNDWORMS

Symptoms of roundworm infestation include weakness, general itching of the body, an uncomfortable swollen abdomen, indigestion, and coughing. Sometimes long pinkish worms come out the nose or mouth or are seen in the stools. Piperazine is the usual chemical medicine given for roundworms, in both animals and people; however, the natural remedies (listed below) may be sufficient to get rid of them.

HOOKWORM

Hookworms enter the body through the skin, usually if a child has walked barefoot over soil that contains the eggs (which have come from feces). The child's feet may start to itch where small worms have gone into the bloodstream. A few days later a cough may begin, when the worms have reached the lungs. The worms may be coughed up and swallowed, causing stomachache, diarrhea, and anemia (symptoms of which are weakness, paleness, and shortness of breath).

A doctor's care should be sought if a child's symptoms suggest hookworm. Stool analysis is the best way to diagnose the condition. Drugs such as TCE (tetrachloroethylene), thiabendazole, mebendazole, and bephenium are usually given. Anemic symptoms often need to be relieved first, to make the child sufficiently healthy to withstand the drugs. (See ANEMIA.)

TAPEWORMS

These parasites usually come from eating meat or fish that has been inadequately cooked. Cysts containing tapeworm eggs, which would have been destroyed by heat, enter the body still alive. The eggs hatch, and tapeworms (which may be yards long) form in the person's intestines; these worms then lay eggs, which are expelled in the person's stool. If the hands are not washed after a bowel movement, the new tapeworm eggs may enter the person's system by mouth and travel on various routes throughout the body. A possible serious result of this is the formation of cysts in the brain, which may bring on weakness, convulsions, or meningitis. Any child with serious symptoms should see a doctor right away. Usually, however, tapeworm infestation causes few symptoms except minor digestive upset. Segments of the worms occasionally crawl out the anus.

Drugs used to kill tapeworms include niclosamide, dichlorophen, and quinacrine.

WHAT YOU CAN DO AT HOME

The following home care measures apply to all worm maladies.
NUTRITION. The child should be given little sugar or fat in his diet, and plenty of raw vegetables (onions, carrots, turnips, and green beans are especially good). Eating several tablespoonfuls of pumpkin seeds every few hours is effective in removing worms. Finely

chopped garlic may be given in salad dressing or in a spoonful of tomato juice juice or soup; children who like the taste can chew and swallow a clove of garlic once or twice a day. Pomegranates, figs, almonds, papaya, and boiled bamboo shoots are also helpful.

HERB TEAS. Slippery elm, fennel, sage, mint, thyme. Wormwood tea is an effective traditional remedy; it tastes abominable, however, and can be toxic—as can the medical worm-killing drugs. Other worm-control measures are usually effective, but if for some reason they do not work, and the parents are strongly opposed to synthetic medications, wormwood tea is an option. The tea is the only effective form of taking his herb; in capsule form it doesn't kill the worms. One teaspoonful of wormwood should be brewed in one cup of boiling water, and taken in spoonfuls throughout the day. Have some fruit juice, dried fruit, or something else very tasty ready to follow the bitter-tasting brew right away.

HOMEOPATHIC REMEDIES. Constitutional homeopathic treatment can strengthen a child's system and help him overcome the ill effects of worms. Find an experienced homeopathic practitioner.

Cina. Child is out of sorts, very irritable, picks his nose, grinds his teeth; and has dark circles around the eyes; distended abdomen.

Santonin. Bad breath, coated tongue, restlessness, and cough at night; may wet the bed.

Teucrium. Child may be restless at night; tingling nose and loss of sense of smell; bad breath; a crawling feeling in the rectum after a bowel movement.

Filix mas or *Kousso.* May be effective for expelling tapeworms.

APPENDICES

HOMEOPATHIC REMEDIES

Following is a list of all the remedies mentioned in the book. Those in capital letters are most commonly indicated or are especially useful in first aid, and may serve as the starting basis for a home remedy kit. Those in regular type are indicated occasionally, and those marked with an asterisk are used more rarely and likely to be needed only for very specific conditions.

ACONITUM NAPELLUS
ALLIUM CEPA
Anacardium orientale
Antimonium crudum
ANTIMONIUM TARTARICUM
APIS MELLIFICA
Argentum nitricum
ARNICA MONTANA
ARSENICUM ALBUM
Baryta carbonica
BELLADONNA
Borax
BRYONIA
CALCAREA CARBONICA
CALCAREA PHOSPHORICA
CANTHARIS
CARBOLICUM ACIDUM
Carbo vegetabilis
Caulophyllum
CAUSTICUM
CHAMOMILLA
CHINA (Cinchona officinalis)
Cimicifuga
Cina
*Cistus canadensis
COCCULUS
Coffea
COLOCYNTHIS
Corallium
Crotalus horridus
Cuprum metallicum
Dioscorea
Drosera
Dulcamara

Equiseteum
EUPATORIUM PERFOLIATUM
EUPHRASIA
FERRUM PHOSPHORICUM
*Filix mas
Fluoric acid
GELSEMIUM
Glonoine
GRAPHITES
HEPAR SULPHURIS CALCAREUM
Hyoscyamus
HYPERICUM
IGNATIA
IPECACUANHA
Iris versicolor
Kali bichromium
Kali bromatum
*Kousso
Kreosotum
LEDUM PALUSTRE
LYCOPODIUM
MAGNESIA PHOSPHORICA
*Mercurius corrosivus
MERCURIUS VIVUS
NATRUM MURIATICUM
Natrum sulphuricum
NUX VOMICA
Petroleum
PHOSPHORUS
Phytolacca
PODOPHYLLUM
PULSATILLA
RHUS TOXICODENDRON
RUMEX CRISPUS

RUTA GRAVEOLENS
*Sabadilla
Sanguinaria
*Santonin
SEPIA
SILICEA
Spigelia
SPONGIA TOSTA
Staphysagria

Stramonium
SULPHUR
SYMPHYTUM
Tabacum
*Teucrium
Thuja
Urtica urens
VERATRUM ALBUM
*Wyethia

Homeopathic Pharmacies

Boericke and Tafel
2381 Circadian Way
Santa Rosa, CA 95407
(800) 876-9505—West Coast
(800) 272-2820—East Coast

Boiron/Borneman
1208 Amosland Rd.
Norwood, PA 19074
(800) 258-8823

Dolisos
3014 Rigel Ave.
Las Vegas, NV 89102
(800) 365-4767

Homeopathic Educational Services
2124 Kittredege St. #40Q
Berkeley, CA 94704
(415) 649-0294

Luyties Pharmacal Company
4200 Laclede Ave.
St. Louis, MO 63156-8080
(800) 325-8080

Standard Homeopathic Pharmacy
210 W. 131st St.
Box 61067
Los Angeles, CA 90061
(800) 624-9659
(800) 992-9659 in California

Guide to Nutrition Supplements

Below are general dosages for commonly supplemented vitamins and minerals, and food sources of these nutrients. Needs for particular nutrients vary drastically from person to person, according to constitution and metabolism. Extra amounts of certain nutrients are often needed during illness and times of stress, or when symptoms of deficiency are apparent. Take care to give all nutrients—especially those for which the infant's and children's doses are not established—in moderation, keeping in mind the child's age and size.

VITAMIN A. RDA—2000 iu for infants; 5,000 iu for teenagers. Supplements: 4,000 to 10,000 iu per day. Huge amounts of Vitamin A can be toxic; if large amounts are taken for therapeutic reasons, use food sources or beta-carotene (which is converted to Vitamin A in the body). Food sources: liver, fish liver oils, egg yolks, carrots, squash, pumpkin, sweet potatoes, lettuce, broccoli, spinach, peaches, apricots, melon, strawberries.

VITAMIN B1. RDA—0.3 mg. for infants; 1.4 mg. for teenagers. Supplements: 5 to 15 mg. per day. Food sources: organ meats, lean meat, yeast, eggs, whole grains, legumes, nuts and berries.

VITAMIN B2. RDA—0.4 mg. for infants; 1.6 mg. for teenagers. Supplements: 5 to 15 mg. per day. Food sources: organ meats, fish, eggs, dairy products, legumes, whole grains, and green leafy vegetables.

VITAMIN B6. RDA—0.3 mg. for infants; 1.8 mg. for teenagers. Supplements: 5 to 15 mg. per day. Food sources: liver, whole grains, yeast, peanuts, blackstrap molasses, corn, soybean, peas, bananas, potatoes, avocadoes, and cabbage.

VITAMIN B12. RDA—0.5 mcg. for infants; 3.0 mcg. for teenagers. Supplements: 5–15 mcg. Food sources: fish, meat, chicken, dairy products, fortified yeast, tempeh, concord grapes, and some seaweeds.

NIACIN. RDA—6 mg. for infants; 18 mg. for teenagers. Supplements: 10–50 mg. Food sources: organ meats, fish, yeast, legumes, whole grains and nuts.

FOLIC ACID. RDA—50 mcg. for infants; 400 mcg. for teenagers. Supplements: 50–400 mcg. Food sources: dark green leafy vegetables, organ meats, asparagus, whole grains, wheat germ, yeast, lentils, lima beans, and citrus fruits.

PANTOTHENIC ACID. RDA—5–10 mg. Supplements: 50–250 mg. Food sources: egg yolks, peanuts, broccoli, cabbage, cauliflower, organ meats, meat, milk, and fruit.

BIOTIN. RDA—150 mcg. for children under four; 300 mcg. for older children and adults. Food sources: egg yolks, filberts, peanuts, mushrooms, cauliflower. Whole grains, liver and organ meats.

CHOLINE. No RDA. Supplements: 50 to 500 mg. per day. Sources of choline are lecithin, egg yolks, milk, corn, soybeans, fish, yeast, organ meats, and beans.

INOSITOL. No RDA. Supplements: 50 to 500 mg. per day. Sources of inositol are lecithin, nuts, fruits, vegetables, yeast, nuts, organ meats, and whole grains.

VITAMIN C. RDA—35–50 mg. for children. Supplements: 100–1,000 mg. per day. Food sources: fresh raw fruits and vegetables, especially citrus, green peppers, parsley, broccoli, cabbage, cauliflower, Brussels sprouts, tomatoes, cantaloupe, strawberries, potatoes and bean sprouts.

VITAMIN D. RDA—400 iu for children (and adults). Supplements: 400 iu per day. Too much Vitamin D can be toxic. If large doses are given for specific deficiency symptoms, use natural sources such as fish oil; avoid the synthetic form. Food sources: fish, egg yolks, liver. "Vitamin D fortified" milk and foods most often contain the synthetic form.

VITAMIN E. RDA—3 iu for infants; 15 iu for adults. This figure was chosen arbitrarily: most persons require amounts much larger than the RDA to stay healthy. Supplements: 50 to 400 iu per day. Vitamin E is found in the oils of soybeans, sunflower seeds, and corn, and also in eggs, nuts, and fish.

CALCIUM. RDA—360 mg. for newborns; 540 mg. for babies under one; 800 mg. ages one to ten; 1200 mg. for teenagers. Supplements: 100–1200 mg. Food sources: dairy products, soy products, egg yolks, broths and stews (made with bones of meat, fish, or poultry), green leafy vegetables, root vegetables, and seeds.

CHROMIUM. No RDA. Supplements: 50–200 mcg. per day. Food sources: black strap molasses, brewer's yeast, whole grains except rye, seafood, meat, nuts, and cheese.

MAGNESIUM. RDA—50 mg. for infants; 150 mg. for children one to three; 350 mg. for teenagers. Supplements: 50–500 mg. Food sources: beans, whole grains, nuts, fruits, green leafy vegetables, and shellfish.

MANGANESE. No RDA. Supplements: 5 to 25 mg. per day. Food sources: whole grains, buckwheat, wheat germ, bran, peas, nuts, fruits (especially blueberries), ginger, and vegetables.

SELENIUM. RDA—50 mcg. for adults. Supplements: 10–50 mcg. Food sources: brewer's yeast, whole grains, seafood, and organ meats.

ZINC. RDA—3 mg. for infants; 10 mg. for children ages one to three; 15 mg. for teenagers. Supplements: 5–25 mg. Food sources: whole grains, pumpkin seeds, wheat germ, brewer's yeast.

GLOSSARY OF HERBS

ALFALFA. The tea is helpful for water retention, digestive and urinary problems.

ALOE VERA. The slippery juice is used on burns and insect bites.

ANISE. The sweet-tasting seed is used to soothe the stomach and urinary tract, to improve appetite and relieve gas, and to help with cramping and spasms.

BARLEY. The water from cooking the grain can be drunk to soothe the throat and digestive tract, or added to baths and skin-washes.

BAY LEAF. Used in cooking or tea, it cleanses the digestive tract; infusions applied externally can help ease muscle aches and skin eruptions; fumes relieve lung and head congestion.

BLACK CURRANT. The leaves in tea are useful in whooping cough.

BLACKBERRY. The fruit, leaf, and root are good for diarrhea.

BUCHU. The leaves in tea are used for urinary problems.

CALENDULA. The flowers are used in tea for anemia, infections, digestive problems; fresh or in tincture for topical use as an antiseptic.

CARAWAY. The seeds are good for digestion, help with colic and bad breath.

CAROB POWDER. The powdered pod of the carob bean is used to control diarrhea; it is also nutritious and often used as a chocolate-subtitute.

CASTOR OIL. For external use, applied to boils; or in a warm cloth placed against the abdomen to relieve constipation or colic.

CATNIP. The tea calms the nerves, soothes the stomach and respiratory tract, and brings on sweat during fever.

CEDAR. The oil is used externally to drive away insects.

CHAMOMILE. The flowers brewed in tea can settle the stomach, calm the nerves, and help cleanse the bowels; applied externally, the infusion soothes skin inflammations and calms irritation of mucous membranes or hemorrhoids.

CHAPARRAL. A strong infusion is used externally for fungus.

CHICKWEED. A wash or poultice applied to the skin is soothing for scrapes, bites, and burns; the tea or fresh herb can act as a laxative and helps with weight loss.

CHICORY. The root is good for digestion and the liver.

CINNAMON. The ground bark freshens breath and helps with indigestion, gas, and bedwetting.

CITRONELLA. The oil is used externally to repel insects.

CLOVE. A temporary antiseptic for toothache (cloves may be bitten, held to the tooth, or used in oil form); the tea relieves sore throat and nausea, and helps digestion.

COFFEE. A strong brew is used at the onset of migraine headaches; stimulates stomach, kidneys, bowels, and gallbladder. Children should only have coffee for medicinal reasons, in small amounts.

COLTSFOOT. The tea is used for asthma, to loosen and bring up mucus.

COMFREY. Used in teas and poultices, the leaves and root help heal broken bones, sprains, and bruises; the tea is good for ulcers, anemia, internal bleeding, heavy menstrual periods, sore throats; poultices, infusions and powders help with burns, wounds, rashes, and skin eruptions.

CORNSILK. In tea is good for urinary problems, especially bedwetting.

CUCUMBER. The fruit eaten raw (in salads) helps eliminate excess water from the body; the juice is good for the intestines, lungs, and skin.

DANDELION. In tea, the root and leaves are good for the liver and digestive system, joint problems, water retention, anemia.

DILLWEED. The seeds, in tea, help with digestion and relieve insomnia; the weed, in tea or salads, is good for cough.

ECHINACEA. A blood purifier, the tea helps the body fight infection, both bacterial and viral; also for digestive problems, anemia, skin eruptions.

ELDER FLOWER. Tea from the dried flowers can relieve cold symptoms, headaches, and bring sweat during fever. (The fresh plant should not be used.)

ELECAMPANE. Tea from the rootstock can ease coughing and aid digestion.

EPHEDRA. The tea is useful in asthma, acts as a stimulant to the liver and urinary organs, and helps relieve migraines.

EUCALYPTUS. The leaves may be made into tea, added to steam and breathed, used in poultices, or rubbed on the chest to clear lung congestion and help soothe asthma and sore throats.

EYEBRIGHT. The tea is used as wash for sore eyes caused by infection or allergy.

FENNEL. The tea can help with anemia and bedwetting; the seeds can be chewed or made into tea to stimulate appetite, help relieve colic, cramps, and gas.

FENUGREEK. The seeds made into tea can help with sore throats, fevers, coughs, lung problems, swollen glands, infections, skin problems.

GARLIC. Raw garlic can fight bacteria and helps remove toxins from the body; reduces mucus in the respiratory tract; good for the heart and arteries; helps expel intestinal worms.

GENTIAN. A tea of leaves and root is good for fever and digestion.

GINGER. Teas or compresses made of the dried or fresh root help relieve gas, soothe sore throat and cough, bring up mucus in asthma, and help bring sweat in fever.

GOLDENROD. The tea is used for urinary problems, whooping cough, arthritis, eczema.

GOLDENSEAL. The powder or tea is used externally as a skin antiseptic; an infusion is used as a gargle to soothe sore throat; small amounts swallowed can help with stomach and liver function.

HOPS. The tea is used for insomnia, restlessness, bedwetting; the flowers are dried and used in herbal pillows.

HOREHOUND. The tea is used for cough, fever, bronchitis, water retention.

IRISH MOSS. In food form or in tea, helps with coughs, improves intestinal function, assists in weight loss.

JUNIPER. The berries, chewed or made into tea, are good for digestive problems; in vapor baths, for chest congestion; the tea can be taken internally and applied to the skin for scabies.

KELP. In the form of tablets or food, good for thyroid function, rich in minerals.

LAVENDER. The tea has sedative action, helps with digestive problems and headaches; soothing as a skin-wash or added to the bath.

LEDUM. Used in tincture form for treating puncture wounds. (Do not use internally; large amounts have caused poisoning.)

LEMON. The juice is used as an antiseptic and astringent; fruit and peel as food or tea are good for liver and skin conditions; source of vitamin C and bioflavonoids.

LEMON BALM. The tea is good for nervous complaints, flatulence, colic, menstrual problems, asthma, nausea, headache, digestive problems.

LICORICE. The root can be chewed or made into tea, for sore throats, menstrual troubles, lung and sinus congestion, allergies; good for the bladder and kidneys.

MARJORAM. Used as a cooking herb or in tea, for indigestion, colic, headache, cough, menstrual cramps, bedwetting; dried and used in an herbal pillow for insomnia; soothing when added to baths.

MULLEIN. The tea is good for coughs, bronchial problems, digestive problems; external applications help with infections, skin problems.

MYRRH. The powder sprinkled on sores can act as a disinfectant; added to steam or burned as incense, fumes help with asthma and cough.

NETTLE. The tea is used for anemia, colds, urinary tract conditions, diarrhea, boils, hair and scalp conditions. (This is the stinging nettle—use it dried or cooked, not fresh.)

OAK BARK (white). The infusion is used as a skin-wash or added to baths for rashes, hemorrhoids, varicose veins; used as a gargle for mouth sores, throat irritations; the tea is used for fever, cough, internal bleeding.

OAT STRAW. The tea helps with bedwetting, kidney and bladder problems, and to strengthen fingernails; used as a wash for skin sores, frostbite, and chilblains.

ONION. Raw and cooked, the root and plant are antiseptic and draw infections, relieve cough, help expel mucus from respiratory and digestive tracts.

ORANGE. Tea made from the peel is good for gas and soothes the stomach; the white inner peel is high in bioflavonids; the fruit and juice are sources of vitamin C.

PARSLEY. The fresh herb, juice, and tea are good for anemia, menstrual problems, coughs, jaundice, asthma; helps fight infection, sweeten breath; used as eyewash.

PENNYROYAL. The oil is good as an insect repellent; the tea makes a soothing wash for irritated skin; taken in small amounts, the tea soothes menstrual cramps.

PEPPERMINT. The tea can relieve nausea, upset stomach, gas pains, headache, and discomfort from fever; added to steam, it clears stuffy nose and sinuses; added to a bath, it soothes itching and joint pains; chewed, the leaves can sweeten breath.

PLANTAIN. The tea can relieve respiratory congestion and digestive troubles; good as a wash or poultice for skin eruptions, itching, burns.

POTATO. Grated raw potato is used as a poultice for infected wounds, blisters, skin eruptions, acne, boils, warts; raw juice is used internally to ease arthritis.

RASPBERRY LEAF. The tea relieves diarrhea and nausea; good for female reproductive organs.

RED CLOVER. The tea is used for allergy and anemia; a blood purifier; the flower and herb are used in poultices for skin irritations, fungal infection, eczema, psoriasis.

ROSE HIPS. The tea is used for anemia, sore throat, coughs, and colds; a source of vitamin C.

ROSEMARY. The tea or herb used in cooking helps relieve indigestion, bedwetting, fatigue and tension; added to steam, it helps clear head and lung congestion; added to baths, it relaxes muscles; the oil can help kill lice and repel most insects. (Do not overuse this herb in teas; large doses can be toxic.)

SAGE. As a cooking herb or tea, it soothes the nervous system, helps ease diarrhea and indigestion; as a wash, it helps itching, rashes, poison oak and ivy, irritated skin.

SHEPHERD'S PURSE. Used as tea or in tincture, it helps control bleeding from wounds, as well as internal bleeding and excessive menstrual flow.

SLIPPERY ELM. The powdered inner bark made into tea, lozenges, or gargle helps sore throats and soothes digestion, relieves diarrhea; the powder applied externally helps skin eruptions and scrapes.

SUMMER SAVORY. Good for digestion; cooked with beans, the herb reduces tendency toward gas; the tea has been said to help in some cases of deafness.

TARRAGON. In tea or as a cooking herb; good for urinary problems, water retention, insomnia, bad breath.

TEA-TREE OIL. The strong-smelling oil has anti-fungal properties.

THYME. As a tea or cooking herb, it helps sore throats, coughs, chest congestion, asthma, diarrhea; added to baths or steam, it helps chest congestion, depression.

TOBACCO. Used as a poultice, the dried leaves draw out venom from insect stings and snakebite. (Not to be used internally; children should not be exposed to the smoke.)

VIOLET FLOWER. The tea and fresh flowers are good for respiratory problems, whooping cough, headache, nervous problems.

WILD CHERRY BARK. The bark made into tea is good for lung problems, cough, and diarrhea. (Do not use the leaves, which are toxic.)

WINTERGREEN. The tea relieves headache, digestive troubles, sore throat; in a wash or rub, soothes skin and sore joints; in steam, helps clear head and lung congestion.

YARROW. A brew made from the root is an effective skin-wash for acne; a tea of the rootstock aids digestion and helps control bleeding.

YELLOW DOCK. The root made into tea works as a blood purifier; helps with digestive problems and anemia; as a wash, soothes skin eruptions.

YERBA SANTÉ. The tea can loosen and bring up mucus in the respiratory tract; good for asthma, coughs, bronchitis, fevers; used as a poultice, a wash, or in baths for sprains, skin irritations, insect bites.

ACUPRESSURE POINTS AND DIAGRAMS

LU 1. A tender point in the indentation below the shoulder end of the collarbone; affects the respiratory tract and skin.

LU 7. The tender point on the undersurface of the thumb-side forearm bone, two of the child's thumb-widths above the palm-side wrist-crease; affects the neck, head, and immune system.

LI 4. The point at the end of the crease between the thumb and index finger; has wide-reaching effects especially on immune response, digestive system, upper extremities, neck and head.

LI 11. A tender point at the thumb-side end of the elbow-crease when the arm is bent; affects the immune system and upper extremities.

LI 20. The tender points where the creases of the cheek meet the nose; help with pain control, depression, allergies, colds, and sinus problems.

ST 12. A "gnawed"-feeling indentation behind the upper middle of the collarbone; affects immune response, digestive and respiratory functions, upper extremities.

ST 25. The tender points two of the child's finger-breadths to either side of the navel; affect the large intestine.

ST 36. A tender point next to the outer side of the big bump at the top of the shin; far-reaching effects include immune and digestive function.

ST 45. The point on the second toe at the edge of the nail bed nearest the foot and the middle toe; good for pain control in toothache.

SP 2. A point on the inner side of the foot at the big toe joint; affects the female reproductive system.

SP 6. A tender point three of the child's finger-breadths above the inner anklebone; along with ST 36, affects immune function; affects the female reproductive system (should not be used during pregnancy).

SP 21. A very tender point below the middle of the armpit, at nipple-level; helps balance body energies; sometimes used for deep or chronic conditions.

HT 3. A tender point on top of the bony bump on the little-finger side of the elbow, at end of crease when the arm is bent; for emotional tension and nervous stress.

HT 7. A point just below the wrist-crease on the little-finger side; calms nervous tension, helps in insomnia.

BL 2. A point just below the bony ridge of the eyebrow, at the end near the nose; helpful in eye problems, headache, sinus conditions, nervousness.

BL 11. The points in the muscles two of the child's thumb-widths to the sides of the vertebra below the bony bump at the base of the neck; helps encourage health of the bones.

BL 25. Points in the muscles just to the sides of the lowest two vertebrae: good for the large intestine, back, and lower extremities.

BL 47. A point in the muscles of the back just above the level of the ridge at the top of the pelvis; affects the female reproductive system, low back, lower extremities.

BL 60. A tender point in the hollow behind the outer anklebone, in front of the Achilles tendon; affects the spine and lower extremities; helps in pain control, depression.

KI 1. A point on the sole between the pads of the ball of the foot; affects the health of the bones, water and mineral balance, hearing, pain control.

KI 3. The tender point just behind the upper rear aspect of the inner anklebone; helps with bones, hearing, hormones, water and mineral balance.

KI 27. A point on the bump found just to the side of the top of the breastbone; used with CV 8 for learning problems and hyperactivity.

P 6. A point in the mid-forearm, three of the child's finger-breadths above the palm-side wrist-crease; for abdominal pain, digestive conditions, depression.

GB 14. A point on either side of the forehead, midway between eyebrow and hairline; for sinus conditions, headache.

GB 20. A tender point in the muscles just below the base of the skull, midway between the central bump on the lower back of the head and the ear tip; for nervous tension, head, neck, sinus conditions.

GB 40. A tender point just below the lower front aspect of the outer anklebone; affects the digestive function, nausea, vomiting, headaches.

LV 3. A tender point midway between the first and second metatarsal bones; affects liver and immune function, allergies, muscle tension.

LV 14. A tender point on the front of the rib cage, midway between the nipple and the lower ribs; affects liver function, allergies, musculoskeletal conditions.

CV 3, 4, 5. Points in the midline of the abdomen, between pubic bone and navel; affect the body's energy and immune function, female reproductive system.

CV 8. The navel (use gentle pressure; hold lightly, don't rub); with KI 27, can affect learning problems, hyperactivity.

CV 12, 13. Tender points midway between the lower tip of the breastbone and the navel; affect digestive function, nausea, vomiting.

CV 22. A point in the notch at the base of the throat, just above the breastbone; good for coughs and asthma.

GV 14. The point at the tip of the big bump in the spine where the neck and upper back meet; affects immune function, endocrine balance, headache.

GV 20. The tender point (a slightly soft spot) at the very top of the head; far-reaching effects include bedwetting, hemorrhoids.

GV 26. The point in the center of the groove between the nose and upper lip; helps in shock, convulsions, unconsciousness.

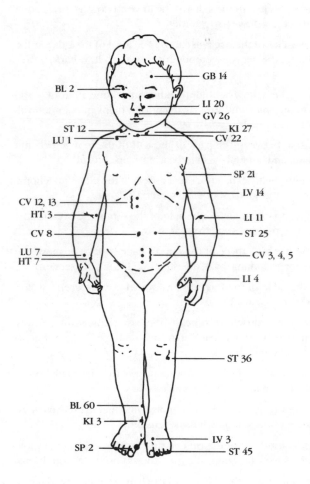

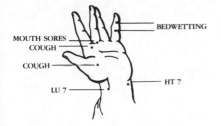

BEDWETTING

MOUTH SORES
COUGH

COUGH

HT 7

LU 7

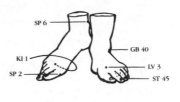

SP 6

KI 1

SP 2

GB 40

LV 3

ST 45

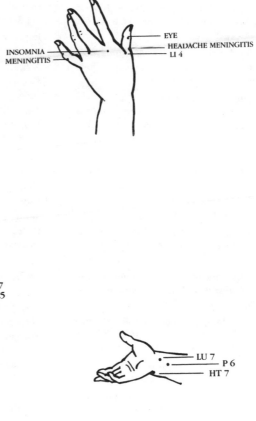

EYE
HEADACHE MENINGITIS
LI 4

INSOMNIA
MENINGITIS

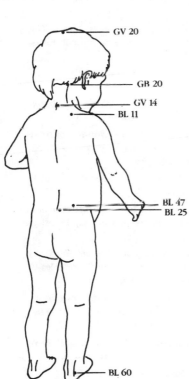

GV 20

GB 20

GV 14
BL 11

BL 47
BL 25

BL 60

LU 7
P 6
HT 7

RECOMMENDED READING

Bach, Edward. *The Twelve Healers and Other Remedies.* London: C.W. Daniel, 1933, 1989.

Blate, Michael. *The Natural Healer's Acupressure Handbook.* New York: Holt, Rinehart and Winston, 1977.

Boericke, William. *Homeopathic Materia Medica with Repertory.* Philadelphia: Boericke & Tafel, 1927, 1982.

Bosco, Dominick. *The People's Guide to Vitamins and Minerals.* Chicago/New York: Contemporary Books, 1989.

Coulter, Harris. *Divided Legacy—The Origins of Modern Western Medicine.* Berkeley, CA: North Atlantic Books, 1988.

Cummings, Stephen, and Ullman, Dana. *Everybody's Guide to Homeopathic Medicines.* 2d ed., rev. Los Angeles: Jeremy P. Tarcher, 1991.

Feingold, Ben. *Why Your Child is Hyperactive.* New York: Random House, 1975.

Ferguson, Tom, ed. *Medical Self-Care: Access to Health Tools.* New York: Summit, 1980.

Harrison, Sheila. *Help Your Child with Homeopathy.* Bath, England: Ashgrove Press, 1989.

Katzen, Molly. *The Moosewood Cookbook* (1977) and *The Enchanted Broccoli Forest* (1982). Berkeley, CA: Ten Speed Press.

Kenyon, Julian. *Acupressure Techniques.* Rochester, NY: Inner Traditions, 1987.

Kirschmann, John D. *Nutrition Almanac.* New York: McGraw-Hill, 1979.

Lust, John B. *The Herb Book.* New York: Bantam, 1983.

Mendolsohn, Robert S. *How to Raise a Healthy Child . . . In Spite of Your Doctor.* Chicago: Contemporary Books, 1984.

Olsen, Kristen Gottschalk. *The Encyclopedia of Alternative Health Care.* New York: Pocket Books, 1989.

Panos, Maesimund, and Heimlich, Jane. *Homeopathic Medicine at Home.* Los Angeles: Jeremy P. Tarcher, 1980.

Pantell, Robert; Fries, James; and Vickery, Donald. *Taking Care of Your Child.* Reading, MA: Addison-Wesley, 1982.

Riggs, Maribeth. *Natural Child Care.* New York: Harmony Books, 1989.

Robertson, Laurel, et al. *The New Laurel's Kitchen.* Berkeley, CA: Ten Speed Press, 1986.

Samuels, Mike, and Samuels, Nancy. *The Well Baby Book.* New York: Summit Books, 1980.

———. *The Well Child Book.* New York: Summit Books, 1982.

Shattuck, Ruth R. *The Allergy Cookbook.* New York: New American Library, 1984.

Smith, Lendon. *The Encyclopedia of Baby & Child Care.* Englewood Cliffs, NJ: Prentice-Hall, 1981.

———. *Feed Your Kids Right.* New York: Dell, 1981.

———. *Improving Your Child's Behavior Chemistry.* Englewood Cliffs, NJ: Prentice-Hall, 1984.

Speight, Phyllis. *Homeopathic Remedies for Children.* Essex, England: Health Science Press: C.W. Daniel, 1983.

Ullman, Dana. *Discovering Homeopathy: Medicine for the 21st Century.* Berkeley: North Atlantic Books, 1988.

Vithoulkas, George. *The Science of Homeopathy.* New York: Grove Press, 1979.

Weeks, Nora, and Bullen, Victor. *The Bach Flower Remedies.* London: C.W. Daniel.

Wright, Jonathan, M.D. *Healing with Nutrition.* Emmaus, PA: Rodale Press, 1984.